GWYNNE. H. DAVIES
N.D.., DO., M.G.O., R.N.T.
Clinical Ecologist

Lighten our Arthritic Darkness

You *don't* have to
'live with it'

To/ Mrs M. J. Maggs
Love and Light
Gwynne H Davies
7. 7. 99.

NIRVANA PRESS

First published in Great Britain by
NIRVANA PRESS
4, Calway Road, Taunton, Somerset. TA1 3EQ

First published 1997

ISBN O 9530817 02

Other titles by author

OVERCOMING FOOD ALLERGIES
THE ALLERGY SUFFERERS
GUIDE THROUGH THE JUNGLE

Printed in Great Britain by
Addicott Printers, Bridgwater, Somerset

CONTENTS

To Rosemarie

ACKNOWLEDGEMENTS

This book is dedicated to a number of people. The first is my dear wife Rosemarie, who has encouraged me, corrected the manuscript, been tolerant with me when I have disappeared to my computer room for hours, and above all, has supported me so admirably in my practice all these years. Without her help and encouragement this book would never have been written. The second is my Secretary Anne Reilly, a tower of strength and my right arm.She too has read the manuscript and made helpful suggestions, I will always be grateful for her support.. To dear Heidi for her comments, constructive criticism, and the injection of encouragement when it was most needed. Last but not least - my patients. They have been an inspiration to me and to them I shall be eternally grateful.Thank you all.

INTRODUCTION

For the last twenty plus years I have treated patients suffering from arthritis. Initially, excluding certain foods such as tomato, wine, red meat and acid foods, because these were the accepted possible causes of the condition. Success was moderate with this approach. However there was enough response to indicate that there was a link between arthritis and what we eat to pursue the subject further. Over the years by discovering the causatory trigger and refining the way of eating to suit the patient the recovery rate is nothing short of staggering.0ut of thousands of patients treated approx 93% responded to diet and supplementation. Mention the association between arthritis and what we eat to a G.P. or Rheumatologist, even in this so called enlightened age, and their response is still a negative one, and they will say that nothing is proven.

I have sent out hundreds of questionnaires to patients I have treated and they are pouring back in to this day. The results speak for themselves - by eliminating allergens the arthritic condition is ameliorated. Out of every hundred responses ninety three report either complete elimination of the condition, or at least, elimination of swelling and reduction in pain levels, without the use of drugs. I have read many books on arthritis and will always be grateful to the authors for they were the pioniers that inspired me to persevere and perfect the procedures I use to such effect today. To these authors I owe gratitude and thanks ;- Giraud Campbell, Dan.D. Alexander, Patricia Byrivers, Jan De Vries, Patrick Holford, John Croft, Malcolm Jayson and Allan St.J. Dixon. M.Hills.

As you will read, it is not easy, and if you are faint hearted, or would rather pop a pill, then please read no further. However if you are sick of being told it is something you will have to live with for the rest of your life, and you know in your heart there has to be another way, then you will be encouraged, heartened, and, I venture to say, excited by what you are about to read and discover.

YOU DO NOT HAVE TO LIVE WITH ARTHRITIS!!!

CHAPTER ONE

LIGHTEN
OUR ARTHRITIC DARKNESS

CHAPTER ONE

Welcome to a world of enlightenment. I have suffered with arthritis and therefore know the nagging, gnawing pain, almost like a deep seated toothache that can keep you awake for hours at night. At times necessitating heaving yourself out of bed and walking around to loosen up, going downstairs so as not to disturb your partner, making a cup of tea, switching on the telly, anything to try and obliterate the pain during the hours of darkness. After treating the condition for twenty years I can tell you here and now, YOU DO NOT HAVE TO SUFFER ARTHRITIS!!!

This is no fairy tale - I am not living in cloud cuckoo land. Providing you are willing to find out what your allergens are and eliminate certain foods you will almost certainly recover. If you have had a long term medical drug treatment, particularly gold, which is the last resort left to Rheumatologists, and alters the blood platelets irrevocably, then it may take considerably longer to obtain relief, but even then you will find a better quality of life immediately and you will be able to look forward to recovery and repair, rather than deterioration.

I am sick and tired of hearing television and radio presenters talking about arthritis being incurable, that you must learn to live with it. Rubbish!!. If in the twentyyears I have been practising I had only helped a handful of patients to recover from this dreadful condition then "they" could be right. But I am not talking about a handful, I am talking about hundreds. All seen on more than one occasion, so, report back, the essential criteria - fulfilled. Many over a period of years, with no sign of a recurrence of symptoms. It is often said by Doctors that the condition is in remission, this is when symptoms subside but flare again at some later date, the only time my patients suffer from a "flare" is when for one reason or another they have strayed from their diet. So gird up your loins, deep breath, say to yourself, I will do it, then you will find **YOU DO NOT HAVE TO LIVE WITH ARTHRITIS!!**

I do not pretend for one moment that it is easy - it most certainly is not. My experience tells me that men find it much harder to keep to a diet than women. Generally speaking this is because men are invariably more sociable and therefore find it hard giving up favourite foods, alcohol etc; The Friday or Saturday night out with the boys is not easy to forego, but there is nothing wrong with going out for the night with the boys and having a fruit juice,is there?- that will prove how strong minded you are. I find that women generally are able to apply themselves much more assiduously and certainly maintain the strict protocol for much longer.I would say this is because they are at home, able to shop for the right foods, and spend more time on the preparation than the average male has. This is why I believe that women have such an important part to play if it is their partner that is suffering. They are able to control the ingestion of food and drink to a great degree, packing up lunches if necessary, and of course encouraging their partner to stick with it and not to give way to temptation.

This could also be an objective judgement on my part - over the twenty years, I have certainly seen far more women than men with the dreaded arthritic condition. Another problem that manifests itself is that most men like their alcohol and are terrible sweet tooth's, I know I am, and this is not easy to give up either. I can think of a couple of occasions where a male patient has said, " I will do everything you tell me, but I will not give up my scotch". I have to say that they have got away with drinking a glass of scotch in the evening with no apparent side effects. However this certainly does not apply to all of us - they are privileged to be lucky enough to escape unharmed, and it is not a recommended course of action.I certainly could not do that without suffering the next day, so particularly in the early stages of the diet do not be tempted to stray from the guidelines.

What is arthritis?. Depending on which book you read, interpretations differ.There are somewhere in the region of twenty eight books on arthritis in circulation at this present time, and each one will tell you something different with regard to recovery. Why I believe this book is so different and should be so helpful, is that it is not based on speculation or because it has worked for a limited number of people, it is based on the clinical evidence of many hundreds of patients over a twenty year period.Only last evening it was on the news that they had found a drug which could help cure cancer, out of the nine persons tested - four responded very well. No doubt that is a good percentage, but what a small sample figure, hardly conclusive to my mind. Always being one to try and simplify things I would say it is a very painful condition affecting the bones and muscles, ligaments, tendons, discs and synovial sacs between large joints. It may be rather cynical of me to adopt this attitude, but I have been convinced for most of my time in practice that the medical profession and scientists love to give things long complicated names to totally confuse the layman. It is amazing when you listen to two Doctors or Specialists talking about your condition, it is as if they were speaking a foreign language. I hope you are the same as me and like to be told what is wrong, in good old basic English, and what you can do to correct it. **You do not have to live with it,** and you will be getting advice on how to overcome it.

The two most common conditions are **osteo-arthritis** and **rheumatoid arthritis**, the first affecting the bone structure and commonly referred to as wear and tear - and the second affecting the musculature and ligamenture. These are fairly straight forward.

Then we get on to the more complicated conditions.

SYSTEMIC LUPUS ERYTHAMATOSUS- a chronic inflammatory disease of connective tissue, affecting the skin and various internal organs - treatment -corticosteroids.

LUMBAR SPONDYLITIS - inflammation of the synovial joints of the backbone.

ANKYLOSING SPONDYLITIS - a rheumatic disease involving the backbone and sacroiliac joints, and sometimes causes arthritis in the shoulders and hips - treatment - analgesics.

REITERS SYNDROME- a disease of men involving diarrhoea , inflammation of the urethra and conjunctiva, and arthritis treatment - steroids.

CERVICAL SPONDYLOSIS - degeneration of the intervertebral discs in the cervical region. Spondilosis can also occur in the thoracic or lumbar region - treatment - non steroidal anti inflammatory drugs (N.S.A.I.D.s.).

OSGOOD SCHLATTERS DISEASE- mostly affecting the young and the knee joints are mainly affected.

PAGETS DISEASE - a chronic disease of the bones, occurring in the elderly and most frequently affecting the skull, backbone, pelvis and long bones. Affected bones become thickened and severe pain ensues - treatment - anti-inflammatory drugs.

SCHEUERMANNS DISEASE - Vertebral osteochondritis found in adolescents. It affects the two rings of cartlilage and bone around the margin of both superior and inferior surfaces of the vertebral body. The condition does not cause general ill health.

POLYARTHRITICA RHEUMATICA - inflammation of many joints. Treatment - N.S.A.I.D.s.

As far as I am concerned these are bone or muscular conditions that mean pain and discomfort and in some cases the distortion of joints - and **YOU DO NOT HAVE TO LIVE WITH IT!!**

So, what is arthritis?. Some mystery disease that affects nearly eight million people in the U.K. Or is it a mystery?. As I hope to show you as we proceed through the book it is not a mystery at all - I call it an allergy reaction. But what is allergy? Here I am quoting from my first book - "Overcoming Food Allergies -1985." The word allergy is often used loosely : people are said to be allergic to anything which does not agree with them. From this has grown the metaphorical or jokey sense in which we speak of a lazy person being "allergic" to hard work. The true meaning of allergy is more precise: it is a condition in which a persons immune system regards an ordinarily harmless substance as a dangerous "invader" and responds to it by producing antibodies, which in their turn give rise to some unpleasant reactions.

Asthma, Eczema, and Hay Fever are perhaps the best known manifestations of an allergic reaction, but in fact the full range of reactions is much more diverse and complicated."

Let me explain in as uncomplicated way as possible the **General Adaptation Syndrome.** Described fully by Professor Hans Selye of Montreal, and adapted and used by **Dr Theron Randolph, M.D**. as the **Specific Adaptation Syndrome** in his book **Human Ecology and Susceptibility to the Chemical Environment.** There are three stages.

STAGE ONE:- Alarm reaction - this could be experienced in a number of ways, but a typical reaction would be a child vomiting when fed cows milk. The mother assumes that this is purely an upset stomach and continues to feed the child cows milk. This initial response, although highly significant, is ignored. The child then moves into the next stage.

STAGE TWO:- This is the stage of adaptation, where although toxins (poisons) are being ingested the body shows only minor reactions and the adrenal glands, situated on top of the kidneys, are able to cope, producing enough adrenaline and cortisone to keep the system stable. Over the weeks, months or years, depending on the amounts ingested, the adrenal glands slowly shrink (atrophy), to the size of a hazelnut, and the toxins begin to win the battle.

STAGE THREE : This is the stage of exhaustion The adrenal glands are unable to cope, the mast cells discharge their histamine and other chemicals, and a severe reaction occurs. This could take the form of an asthma attack, epileptiform manifestation, skin rash, or arthritis,or childhood growing pains!!

It is in these circumstances, when a toxin is ingested, that a pancreatic maladaption takes place and "triggers" the whole process. In the case of arthritis, it is my hypothesis that the Kinin, (a pain transmitting hormone), breaks down into Bradikinin and this is the instigatory cause of the arthritic inflammation or deterioration.

What will become clear to you as you read on, is that by treating the condition in this way and discovering the "allergy', eliminating it completely, and keeping to a strict way of eating, the condition is ameliorated.

There have been numerous books on Arthritis written over the years, where putting the authors partner on a special diet and avoiding certain foods, has eliminated the condition. Marvellous, I am not knocking that approach, it is just that I believe it is much more individualistic than that, as each person reacts in their own way, but the clinical evidence I have amassed over the last twenty or so years has convinced me that there is an overall pattern observed, and if we adopt that pattern initially, **most** people will respond.

THE MECHANISM OF ALLERGIC REACTION

I will now attempt to clarify the mechanism of allergic reaction. A person who is allergic will react to his or her allergen in rather the same way as healthy people react to a possibly dangerous micro-organism or to a poison. In both cases the defence mechanism of the body is stimulated by the presence of an antigen (living or organic matter foreign to our own proteins). Viruses and bacteria are antigens, and, so are normally less dangerous substances like foods, pollens etc; Our defences depend on lymphocytes (white cells), whose function it is to distinguish between harmful and innocuous antigens.

When white cells come across an antigen, which looks as though it may cause harm to the body, they produce antibodies: the antibodies combine with the antigen and render it harmless. Even in a healthy person it may take several days for the white cells to produce enough antibodies to inactivate the antigen, but once the antigen has been dealt with the body has long lasting protection against it.

This is the reason why most people only suffer from infectious diseases like measles or chickenpox once in their lives. When the virus attacks for a second time there are antibodies at hand to dispose of it quickly. This is the general idea behind vaccination: you are given a minute dose of an antigen which is not strong enough to give you the disease, but is strong enough to cause the white cells to produce the antibodies and protect you.

In an allergy-prone person the white cells react to a harmless anitigen as if it were an invader. No one is really clear as to why this should happen, although evidence indicates that it may well be a hereditary problem. Allergies do tend to run in families, and there is some evidence that allergic people lack a particular type of white cell which controls the production of antibodies.

It happens in far too many cases where children have been weaned off the breast too early in their lives, laying them open to infection at a later stage.

This often reveals itself as an allergy to dairy products. This tendency is further complicated by the fact that we have not one mechanism for allergic reaction but several.

What usually happens?

The arrival of an antigen stimulates the production of large quantities of white cells, and no particular reaction is noticeable. The antibodies, which then have nothing to do but wait for the next invasion attach themselves to tissue cells known as mast cells. A mast cell contains a number of natural chemicals, histamine being the most plentiful. The function of the histamine is to increase the flow of fluids in and out of blood vessels, to control the production of fluid in the mucous glands, and to make muscles in the internal organs contract. These events are happening all the time and are regulated automatically by the body without any conscious thought on our part. Once a mast cell has been coated with antibodies it is liable to become excited: the next dose of an antigen stimulates the antibodies into action and the mast cell reacts by releasing its stock of histamine and other chemicals.

What happens then?

That depends on where the mast cells are located. We are compartmentalised like a ship, and if the mast cells affected are in the head, then the outcome may well be a streaming nose (chronic rhinitis),asthma, gut dysbiosis(diarrhoea or constipation) or a skin eruption. Our biological structures are all as different as our finger prints, so the problem facing a practitioner specialising in allergic reactions, (a Clinical Ecologist), are enormous and very complicated. A good analogy would be that of crossing a minefield. I issue new patients with a booklet to help them in the initial stages called "The Allergy Sufferers Guide Through The Jungle". It was therefore, only after a great deal of research and correlation of evidence that I have been prompted to write this book and my previous book and booklets.

I hope that has helped you to understand the link between allergy and arthritis.

Let me for a moment try and bring these entities together. Remember this is my hypothesis, but one that has proved to be correct in the assessment and successful treatment of arthritics for over twenty years. As I have mentioned previously I believe the cause to be - a pancreatic malfunction. The inability of the pancreas to recognise the enzymes in certain foods, "invaders", and causes a release of mast cell toxins which then permeate the system. Insidiously as with osteo-arthritis, and in many cases, instantly with rheumatoid type reactions. In the Lipase, Amyláse, Trypsinogen phase of pancreatic function we should break down the enzymes and produce Enterokinase or Enteropeptinase in the duodenum, this then produces healthy cellular function. This is when the breakdown occurs and Kinin and Bradikinin are produced - a breakdown in the normal processes - and pain and discomfort ensue.

Kinin is one of a group of naturally occurring polypeptides that are powertul vasodilators, which lower blood pressure, and cause contraction of smooth muscle. The kinins bradikinin and kallidin are formed in the blood by the action of proteolytic enzymes (kallikreins) on certain plasma globulins (kininogens). Kinins are not normally present in the blood, but are formed under certain conditions; for example when tissue is damaged, or when there are changes in the pH and temperature of the blood. They are thought to play a role in inflammatory response.

In his book, Allergies - Your Hidden Enemy, Dr Theron Randolph M.D. (the alma mater of Clinical Ecology) devotes a whole chapter to arthritis, and the association between this condition and food substances and chemical susceptibility. The first definitive work was published by Doctor Michael Zeller in 1949 and titled Rheumatoid Arthritis - Food Allergy as a Factor. These men were the pioniers of clinical ecology and its use in the relief of debilitating diseases.

Since the 1920's medical practitioners have been recording individual maladaptive reactions to foods and chemicals, observed as emerging during controlled systematic test exposures.

The tests I have carried out for the past twenty plus years is conclusive evidence that the pancreas, the INSTIGATORY endocrine-exocrine organ of the body, gives us the key to relieving the many debilitating conditions prevalent in society today. Arthritis in all its guises - and they are numerous, is an inflammatory condition.

At this point I would like to quote from a book that has been very important to me, understanding the psychology of disease. It is called " Brain Allergies - The Psychonutrient Connection", Kalita and Philpott - both M.D.'s.The following is a quote from that book.

"The `hard way' to to discover truth need not be the only one. We must always keep in mind that the greatest enemy of any science or any discovery of truth is a closed mind. Accordingly, we should seek the courage to ask impertinent questions which will shake our complacency, challenge our minds, and to look dèeper into the farthest reaches of the great mystery of the human body. Then and only then will we be able to accept truth at face value".

It is very easy to become complacent and say aren't I a clever lad, and why doesn't the rest of the world agree with me?. By introducing case histories from my patients it could be said that I could be accused of self glorification. I hope and pray that you will not consider that to be the case. The inclusion of case histories is to give you, the reader, the opportunity to share with fellow sufferers what you are going through. I am sure that those of you who suffer with arthritis will identify with at least one of the cases. The first one is very typical of what does happen and how you too can help ameliorate your condition.

Mrs D. T. Isle of Wight.

"It was a Wednesday afternoon middle of May 1978 when I started to feel poorly. It started with a headache at the back of my head, which eventually came up over the top and I thought I had caught a heavy cold. I went to bed early and awoke the next morning with fingers as big as sausages and very painful. On the Friday I was feeling quite poorly, and in pain, so my husband decided to ring a specialist for a private appointment. He said he would see me on the Saturday morning. He went into my past health history and I told him that at the age of twelve I had rheumatic fever. After an examination he referred me to the local hospital for blood tests and asked me to come back the following Wednesday for the results. We did, and my husband and I were absolutely shattered when he told us I had Rheumatoid Arthritis and would be in a wheel chair within three years. We walked away absolutely devastated but my husband Ron said to me "if they think I am going to wheel you around in a wheel chair after the hard working life we have had they have another think coming, we are going to fight this thing".

The doctor had even told my husband we would have to sell the business because I would not be able to cope. So the fight began. I went back to my own G. P. and he then told us he was putting me on Opren, my husband asked him what the side effects would be, "Oh!" he said, "not much, she may get indigestion or a rash or she won't be able to go out in the sunlight". As I had never suffered these things and I love the sun I refused to take this drug wasn't I the lucky one ! !.

So, my husband decided to take me to Harley Street for a second opinion, but there I was told more or less, "hard cheese, you will have to learn to live with it". I had attended physiotherapy sessions Mon/Wed/Fri which left me in agony on Tues/Thurs/ Sat/Sunday, so I decided I would not go, and by now the pain was all over my body. We had a Post Offce and I found I could not count the notes very well and it was very painful to tear the stamps, but I plodded on.

Every so often I had to attend the Rheumatoid Clinic where the Specialist was very off hand and not a bit sympathetic, so one day the nurse said to me, "how are you today Mrs T?", I had to tell her that I felt very poorly, I pained everywhere and there was very little let up, and I am afraid I was a little down that day.

Oh! let me go back to the Christmas, because this is now February 1979 and we had gone to my daughter Gillian's for Christmas, and on Boxing Day she held open house for all my old friends. I was sitting on the settee and one of my friends asked Gillian where I was and Gillian told her I was on the settee, and her reply was, "not that little old lady?". Now I am anything but a little old lady but that is just what I looked like. A few days later after we got home I had a letter from that friend with a card enclosed and it said,

"Doreen go and see this man, you will never regret it".

Now I will go back to my visit to the specialist. The nurse said I want you to get undressed Mrs T because he has never examined you properly. I was called in to his office feeling very very poorly. He was sitting at his desk writing and did not even look up, even when I said "good morning", he just said "what can I do for you". I told him I was feeling very poorly and his answer then sent me in to floods of tears. He said "You are like my car standing outside, you need all new spare parts and I cannot give them to you. You seem to think you can get better on hard work and brown bread, but it will not work and you have not attended physiotherapy, in fact I do not wish to see you again". I was devastated and told him that I did not wish to see him again either.

When I got back to the Post Offce my girls who worked for us told my husband to "go upstairs and sort me out". That was when he rang the number on the card my friend sent and made an appointment to see Gwynne Davies.

I saw Gwynne Davies in February 1979 and he informed me it was a pancreatic malfunction causing the problem and I was producing a pain transmitting hormone called kinin, this was breaking down in to bradikinins, tiny razor edged crystals and these were attacking the joints and creating the inflammation. He tested me for my allergies and told me to avoid all milk products, oranges, tomatoes, rhubarb, gooseberry, strawberry, beetroot, spinach, peppers and radish. Peel apples and wash all fruit thoroughly. He then put me on a strict arthritic diet and within three weeks I noticed a decrease in the pain and started to improve. I am now free of pain and stiffness and providing I do not stray from the straight and narrow I feel fine.

To summarise, in May 1978 I was told I would be in a wheel chair within three years, I started the treatment with Gwynne Davies in 1979, it is now sixteen years on and I am 68 years of age and I can give many a 40 year old a run for their money'. So, you see, **YOU DO NOT HAVE TO LIVE WITH ARTHRITIS!!**

I am often asked by patients which food is the biggest culprit?. As I pointed out earlier, there have been many books published on arthritis, and therefore there have been differing opinions as to the major culprits, many of these pure hypothesis. What I am trying to do in this book is to tell you what has worked so well in a clinical situation, treating not a handful, but thousands of patients. I have to be honest and say the biggest culprit is milk.

Living in a rural area like Taunton in Somerset, with hundreds of dairy farmers and dairy farmers wives as patients you can imagine, that statement goes down like a lead balloon, but it is a fact. Out of the thousands of arthritic patients that have consulted me over the years at least 90% are allergic to milk and associated products. Certainly where osteo arthritis is concerned milk is always the major culprit. Where rheumatoid arthritis is concerned then milk is usually the basic causatory trigger but exacerbated by so called acid foods.

I am often challenged on the use of the word allergy. Because it is not a true immunological response it is not correct to use the word allergy, we should use hypersensitivity, but we are not here to split hairs. The main thing as far as I am concerned is that patients understand that they cannot tolerate dairy products. Allergy is a word most people understand and can come to terms with. Whatever you call it - hypersensitívity or allergy, the results are the same, pain, stiffness and swelling. So in a moment let us look in more depth at milk,explained on page 15, and the possible reasons we cannot tolerate it. I often say, "it is simple, a cow has four stomachs and we only have one, so how can we digest it". What is a cows natural diet?. It eats grass.

Needless to say there are differing viewpoints as to why milk is so deleterious to our health generally. Certainly the Milk Marketing Board as it used to be called will disagree with these assumptions, but one would expect them to. They are in the business of getting you, the public, to drink as much as possible to make a profit for their customers.

When you think of the millions of pounds already spent, and still being spent on advertising this product it is not surprising the public have fallen for it. **MILK IS GOOD FOR YOU!! DRINK A PINTA DAILY !! YOU NEED MILK TO GET CALCIUM AND BUILD HEALTHY BONES !!**

What a load of nonsense that all is. Admittedly we all need calcium and other minerals to build healthy bones, nails, teeth and hair, but milk is not the way to get it. Have you ever seen a native of Africa or an Eskimo with bad nails, teeth, hair or bones?. I have not, unless they have been in this country for some time and have become Westernised in their dietary habits.

What have we done to our milk over the years ?.

HOMOGENIZING - We are told that this is a good process and very necessary, it permits milk to stand around longer without going sour. It prevents milk and cream from separating, great!!

We do not have to go to the enormous trouble of shaking the bottle each time, very tiring. But there is a price to pay for saving our muscle strength and making less trips to the local shop. The process of homogenisation consists of putting milk under high pressure and elevated temperatures. This changes the raw protein in milk and makes it less nutritional. It destroys an enzyme called phosphatase which is necessary for the utilisation of calcium and phosphorous. It destroys some of the valuable B-Vitamins and some of the C -Vitamins.

Right up until the early 1900's milk was a whole food. It was not skimmed, boiled, powdered, condensed, pasteurised or homogenised.

I know, yes, you are quite right, occasionally it was certified. But what did that mean?. It was a means of ensuring that through controlled feeding conditions the milk was nutritious, fresh, and hygienic. BUT IT WAS NOT PROCESSED !!

You do not need to be an Einstein to see that the many hundreds of changes that have taken place with the production, feeding,and de-naturisation of pastureland, the precious "balance of nature" has been destroyed, and the consequences of absorption within our own bodies affected.

There was a time when I thought that raw milk was the best thing for patients. In other words straight from the cow, no homogenisation or pasteurisation. This view has changed over the years for many reasons, but the main reason being that 95-98% of arthritics tested are allergic to it. Thankfully there is an alternative, goat or sheep milk, and let us put this bogey to bed about these alternative milks not being so good for you. From a nutritional point of view, ewes milk is the most concentrated milk food. Typical differences in the energy value of the three milks are expressed here in kilocalories (kcal) as well as in the modern terminology of kijoules (kj), (1 calorie = 4.184 joules.).

	kca	lkj
Sheep	102	426
Goat	71	296
Cow	65	272

These figures were taken from" Practical Sheep Dairying" by Olivia Mills - Thorsons 1982.

Another good reference for anyone interested in following tables of comparisons should refer to" Health Hazards of Milk", D. L. J. Freed, Bailliere Tindall,1984. I can assure you that the calcium levels between them is so little it is not worth considering.

You will appreciate of course that goat and sheep milk are full fat, and in the early stages of the diet when the major detoxification is taking place, and the poor old liver has to work overtime, I recommend that you dilute them with 50% water.This also saves money of course.This at least gives the liver a chance to decongest and absorb proteins more readily, and the fats of course. In the leaflet I give to patients outlining the dangers of mìlk consumption, the following are pertinent.

The milk of any species was designed for one purpose only, to feed its young. Human beings are the only creatures on this earth that drink the milk designed for another species, and we continue to do so all our adult lives, never weaning ourselves off it. Can you imagine a calf, kid, or lamb trying to continue feeding from its parent, it would be kicked off and encouraged to eat grass as nature intended. What do we do to the poor old cow?. We encourage it to continue pumping out milk every day of its life and for what purpose?; To feed human beings who are continually bombarded by radio, television and advertising, plus the medical profession, to drink milk because it is good for you. If you saw the state of the bone structure of some of my patients you would soon realise that it is not gooc for you at all, and far from feeding the bones, cows milk actually depletes the bone structure.

The enzymes we need to break down and digest milk are renin and lactase. By the age of four, many of us lose the ability to digest lactase because we can no longer synthesise the digestive enzyme lactose. This lactose intolerance results in diarrhoea, flatulence and bowel or stomach cramps. Some 90% of adult Asian and black people, and 20% of Caucasian children are lactose intolerant.

The level of protein in cows milk is 300 times higher than in human breast milk, which is predominantly made up of the protein lactalbumin, which is easily digestible by babies. Nature has designed the milk of each animal species specifically to meet the needs of its young. Casein is intended to be broken down by the four-stomach digestive system of baby cows. In human stomachs it coagulates and forms large tough, dense, diffcult to digest curds. When the protein of another animal is introduced into the body, it may cause an allergic reaction, (Journal of Allergy, 41 : 226,1968.), the most common symptoms of which are chronic runny nose, persistent sore throat, hoarseness, bronchitis and recurrent ear infections.**THE MUCOUS MEMBRANES LINING THE JOINTS AND LUNGS CAN BECOME SWOLLEN OR INFLAMED, CONTRIBUTING TO RHEUMATOID ARTHRITIS AND ASTHMA.**
Highlighted to bring the point home to you.

As I have mentioned already, milk is touted as a great natural source of calcium, and we are told to ingest calcium to prevent osteoporosis or thinning of the bones. In fact, eating dairy products can increase the rate at which calcium is lost from the bones and so hasten osteoporosis.

As well as being high in calcium, dairy products are also high protein foods. If we have too much protein in the diet from milk products or any other source, such as meat, fish, or eggs, the body has to get rid of the excess. To do this the kidneys must lose calcium as they cleanse the blood of excess waste, a process known as protein induced hypercalcuria.(J.Nutr III;553,1981; Trans NY Acad Sc 36;333,1974; Am Clin Nutr, 27; 916m,1974).

People in the United States and Scandinavia consume more dairy products than anywhere else in the world, yet they have the highest rate of osteoporosis (Clin Ortho Related Res,152;35,1980). This fact emphasises the threat of excessive protein in the diet and suggests that dairy products offer no protection against osteoporosis, probably due to the high content of milk. (Am J Clin Nutr,41;254,1985).

The body's ability to absorb and use calcium depends on the amount of phosphorous in the diet. The higher the calcium/phosphorous ratio the less bone loss takes place and the stronger the skeleton, providing the intake of protein is not excessive. The foods which contain higher calcium/phosphorous ratios are fruit and vegetables. Low fat milk is no better for you either, remember - a little does do harm!. Low fat milk contains one per cent butter fat and the full compliment of allergy inducing milk protein. ! !

Getting bored with all this talk of the dangers of ingesting milk?. I hope not for there is more to come yet, but let us break for a moment the intensity of the subject and -lighten your darkness - by quoting another case history from someone who is allergic to milk.

Mrs D. S. Waterlooville, Hants. 8-10-95.

"Before I consulted Gwynne Davies my condition had deteriorated a great deal since first visiting my G.P. and a Rheumatologist, who could offer no hope of improvement, and would prescribe stronger drugs. I was sent to the local hand clinic of the local hospital who gave me hand splints to help straighten my fingers. I had reached a stage where I could not hold a newspaper without a lot of pain in my hands and forearms. I could not lift a bag of sugar, a kettle, or make the beds because I could not bear the weight on my hands. I found it impossible to turn the ignition key of the car, and was so tired I needed a rest every afternoon which was totally out of character. I seldom could take a bath because I could not get out, neither my wrists or my knees were strong enough to lift me, and I could only walk a short distance.

Within a few days of starting the treatment recommended by Gwynne Davies, I lost most of the pain, and within two weeks there was a marked improvement in my health. At the beginning I weighed about 11 stone 10 lbs, I am now 10 stone. After twenty one months I am a different person, much more active both physically and mentally, and I play an active part in the community again.

I can now run a home, drive a car, and take my dog and my grandchildren for long walks. I have taken up swimming for the first time, and as a keen horsewoman I am considering riding again. It has been a wonderful cure, and every day I give thanks for the skills of Gwynne Davies".

So you see, **YOU DO NOT HAVE TO LIVE WITH ARTHRITIS!!**

Now to return to the thorny subject of milk. Added to the list of problems already mentioned there is the inherent problem of humans consuming milk designed for baby cows. We can also add a host of "unnatural" ones. Cows milk contains the accumulated pesticides that have been sprayed on to the grain to feed the cattle, and the pastureland, and the female hormones given to cows to increase milk production and body fat. Some milk has also been shown to contain trace metals and radioactivity at levels higher than those permissible in drinking water.

Some 20% of milk producing cows in America are infected with leukemia viruses which, because the milk is pooled when collected, infects the whole milk supply. What a scenario! ! These cancer inducing viruses are resistant to being killed by pasteurisation and have been recovered from supermarket supplies(" Medical World News",16 May,1969). Can it really be coincidence that the highest rates of leukemia are found in children aged 3 -13 years of age, who consume the most milk products, and in dairy farmers who, as a profession have the highest rates of leukaemia in any group??. I think not.

I certainly do not wish to bore you with a book full of statistics. Apart from anything else they can be massaged in such a way as to show what you wish to show. But at the same time I have to look at the Clinical evidence, the proof of the pudding as it were. This speaks volumes and I hope to show this throughout the book.95-98% of all arthritic patients I have treated, and they run into many thousands, have been allergic to cows milk. What is even more important is that they have all reaped benefit by eliminating it from their diets. As I said earlier it is contrary to the chapter on arthritis in my last book, Overcoming Food Allergies, Ashgrove Press,1985. The evidence was not available or as clear cut as it is now, and if this book is going to help those suffering from the dreaded arthritis or osteoporosis, then this evidence must be made available, times change and statistics alter.

You will hear me repeating time and time again throughout the book, do not think by just eliminating milk you have solved the problem. The plain and simple fact is you have not. It is much more complicated than that. The elimination of all dairy products from ones diet is no easy matter. You will need to check labels at all times. I am asked so many times by patients, "is it alright when I am out if I have just a little?". My reply is always the same "No, you might just as well have a bucketful!!" I certainly know when I have had something wrong. My hands are stiff and the skin sensitive, and my hip and knee hurt. One lady came back for a second appointment and showed me her hands and the fingers were like small sausages. "What on earth have you been doing I asked". "Well I find it difficult to believe but a few nights ago I went out for a meal with friends and had some butter in a sauce, surely it can not be that?". The answer is of course, yes it was just that. After ten days the toxins had cleared again and she was fine.

Milk really does lurk in the most unlikely places. Who would think that if you had a gravy made with Bovril that you were having milk. But you are, there is lactose in it. Who would think when you accepted a wine gum and ate it, that you were ingesting lactic acid, but you are and it is there in the small print, and sometimes very, very small print.

Oh! I can't have butter, never mind I will have margarine. No you cannot! ! Margarines contain lactic acid and whey, both milk derivatives. There are alternatives at, present they are available in health shops. I believe it will not be long before the margarine manufacturers will be producing non-hydrogenated margarines as a matter of course. You will no doubt be aware from television and newspapers that a war has gone on for years, with each side arguing the merits of their own product, quite understandably of course. So, which margarines can you have that are safe -

GRANOSE RED LABEL, GRANOVITA, WHOLE EARTH, VITAQUELLE. These are all non-hydrogenated margarines, with no trans-fatty acids and much better for you, and can be used for cooking. Having said that, for pastry making when you are fit and well enough, then TOMOR from the supermarket is the one of choice. It is a Kosher margarine.

Help! that means I cannot have cheese!. Not true, you can, and what is more they are delicious, I will try and list some of the most popular ones. CHEVRES, HALUMI, EFTAKI, FETA, PECORINO, MANCHEGO, CABRALES, ROCQUEFORT plus many other goat and ewes milk cheeses.. A choice selection for anyone. ARF Vegetarian cheese. ARF means Animal Rennet Free, some health shops will tell you that this is not permissible if you are allergic to dairy because it is made with cows milk. This is not true either. I have tested patients for fifteen years on Vegetarian cheese, and providing you do not cook it or heat it any way, and thereby not reducing the enzymatic structure back to milk it is perfectly safe. So do not cook Vegetarian cheese! ! The difference between ordinary cheddar cheese and vegetarian cheese is the curdling agent - rennet. To make a thousand gallons of milk into cheese you need 4ozs of rennet. Does that not make your mind boggle? Avoid soft and red coloured vegetarian cheeses.

We are talking about 1 in 100,000 parts dilution - a 10 millionth part! !

That is so microscopic it is not true, and yet the reaction to every patient tested is the same, ordinary cheese - total failure. Vegetarian cheese - total success. So the moral of that is please do not let anyone convince you "that a little bit wìll not hurt you! !". They are not the ones that are going to suffer next day, and possibly for several days afterwards.

Are there alternative milks?. Of course there are. Goat milk, sheep milk and soya. I have to be honest and say that I do not like soya milk as it leaves a dry nutty taste in the mouth, but hundreds of patients tell me they quite like it in preference to goat or sheep. We are all individuals thank goodness, and all our tastes are different; what a dreary old world this would be were that not so. I have certainly found that sheeps milk does not vary very much at all in taste or texture, but goat milk does. So if you are not happy with the one you have tried, do shop around until you find one you do like. Both goat and sheep milk have a high fat content and I certainly advise my patients to water it down by 50% to start with, then try full strength later if they feel like it. Do not put babies on it without advice from a practitioner. There are several organic soya milks on the market, PLAMIL,GRANOSE, PROSOBEE ETC;.

Do not use UHT or Pasteurized goat or sheep milk if possible.

DANGER!!! BEWARE!!! If you have a milk allergy avoid the following:-

LACTOSE, LACTASE, LACTIC ACID (E270), CASEIN, WHEY, SKIMMED MILK.

The undermentioned products can, and frequently do contain milk in one form or another. It will drive you mad shopping for approximately three weeks while you read all the labels, and get used to which products are safe, but you must check! !

Baking Powder. Biscuits. Bakers bread (sliced packet loaves). Bavarian cream.

Blancmange. Boiled salad dressings. Bologna. Butter. Buttermilk. Butter sauces.

Cakes. Chocolates. Chocolate or Cocoa drinks or mixtures. Cream. Creamed foods.

Cream sauces. Cheeses. Curds. Custards. Doughnuts. Eggs scrambled. Escallop dishes. Foods prepared au gratin. Food fried in butter,(fish,poultry, Beef, pork, ham, bacon, veal,). flour mixtures, fritters, gravies. Hamburgers. Hash, turkey breast, turkey roll, some frozen turkey, some chicken breasts. Hard sauces. Ice creams. Mashed potato. Malted milk. Ovaltine. Meat loaf. Cooked sausages. Omelletes. Oleomargarines. Pastry crust. Popcorn. Prepared food mixes for biscuits,cakes, muffins, pancake, pie crust, waffles, puddings. Rarebits. Salad dressing. Sherberts. Souffles.Some Soups. Sweets. Junket.Some lowfat crisps.

This list is a guide. Manufacturers do change the contents of their products frequently, so, be on your guard and make vigilance your password. A classic example of this was several years ago when I advised patients to use "Outline" margarine as it did not contain lactose, I then started getting phone calls from all over the country from patients complaining that many of their old symptoms had returned. When contacted, Van Den Bergh the manufacturers had decided, in their wisdom, to add lactose and call it " NEW

Outline". When the patients were advised of this and they removed it from their diet, their symptoms soon disappeared.

You will remember earlier I mentioned Pork, Ham, Bacon, and Veal, as being wrong to eat. This is because to this day whey is used to feed pigs and whey is a milk by-product.

However if you know a butcher that can supply non whey fed pork then you are allowed to eat this. Do please note that because it may be stated that it is organic pork, this does not mean it is not whey fed, it invariably is. It really is amazing how many patients say, " I cannot eat pork it makes me ill". On the pages that will follow recommending the foods to eat, you will see meat mentioned, this is an endeavour to balance out the diet as much as possible. It really is predominantly fruit and vegetables, and if at all possible eat organic food. If you can grow your own without the use of pesticides and sprays then so much the better.

What is more you will certainly notice the taste is so different. We are fortunate here in Taunton as we have a butcher Mr Dennis Bates, Select Meat Co, Bath Place, Taunton, Somerset who specialises in conservation grade meats. and the taste is reminiscent of how meat used to taste! We also have very close at hand two dedicated people, Anne and Kieron McGrath, who take organic rearing to its optimum. Their rare breeds meat and poultry has to be tasted to be believed. The Bell and Bird Table, Runnington, Wellington, Somerset.

When I tell you that their meat and poultry is used in some of the top hotels in the country you will realise just how special it is. Needless to say you cannot just turn up and buy it, orders do have to be made in plenty of time. During the war, and that gives my age away, but those of you who remember those days will remember how bacon used to cook, simmering away gently in the frying pan with that special smell, and the taste! ! Nowadays the bacon spatters all over the kitchen, the smell is not at all appetising, and the taste is moderately acceptable. What is more, when you cook organic pork the crackling actually crackles!!. In my previous book I recommended the ingestion of organ meats as being good for you, I no longer believe this to be true and recommend that unless things change dramatically over the next five years or so do not eat organ meats ! !.

A question I am often asked is "how long do I have to keep to the diet?". The answer of course - for ever if you wish to stay free of swelling and pain. I have kept to it for twenty years now and have no intention of detracting from it. If you were born with a pancreatic malfunction, which produces a pain transmitting hormone bradykinin, then until such times as someone gives you a replacement you keep to the straight and narrow. As I have said before, it is straight and at times when friends and relatives are filling their faces with "goodies"!!, it is very narrow. However they are not the ones that suffer with the pain or the swelling, so you do not listen when in all sincerity they say, "Oh! go on a little can't hurt surely". But we know different don't we. I suffer from psoriasis as well as arthritis, and if I detract from the straight and narrow, which thankfully does not happen deliberately or very often, then my hands become stiff and swollen and the psoriasis will appear somewhere on my body. So I learnt many years ago it just is not worth it. I am quite sure that once you have experienced the joy of moving freely again, without pain or swelling then you too, will not wish to stray.

In the majority of cases the condition has not flared up overnight, it has been one of slow but sure deterioration. That is not to say that some patients with rheumatoid arthritis report that they went to bed with no pain at all, in the early hours of the morning they were woken up with awful pains in the joints, and in most cases swollen joints too. Very often there is reddening and heat can be felt emanating from a particular joint or joints. Quite sensibly the patient reports to the G.P. and invariably one of two things happens, the patient is prescribed an anti inflammatory drug NSAID, of which more in the next chapter.

A blood sample is then taken and sent to the laboratory and the results are confirmed within fourteen days. It really is amazing how these results vary. Many are told that the result is positive and to take the NSAID's, and if the pain gets worse come back and have something stronger, or at worst you may need operative procedures. What an outlook, abandon hope all ye that enter these portals. Others are told that the results are negative so there is nothing further that can be done.

Now let us take a few salient points from that last paragraph. The joint can be swollen and reddened and heat can be felt emanating from it. Certainly in the case of hands and feet distortion of these limbs can be seen in a comparatively short space of time, this is invariably rheumatoid arthritis and is extremely painful. It really is quite amazing how many patients have related the above to me and presented with the obvious symptoms and yet they are told the tests are negative, we do not know what the condition is, it could get worse, and you will have to live with it.

I recall vividly, something like ten years ago, a young lady in her thirties consulted me with her husband, she came from Bridgwater and her hands were distorted and swollen, the pain was excruciating and preventing her from sleeping properly. She presented herself to her G.P. three times, blood samples were sent off and returned as negative, to be told by her doctor that she did not have rheumatoid arthritis.

What did she have then?. Surely the doctor had been in practice long enough to recognise the condition without the need of blood tests. I informed her that I had seen enough of the condition over the years to recognise it as rheumatoid arthritis and I would be treating her as such. On testing she proved hypersensitive to, have you guessed yet?, of course you have - dairy products!

There were others, apple skin, tomato, rhubarb, gooseberry, strawberry, beetroot, spinach, peppers, radish, and because of the rheumatoid involvement she was told to blanch her onions and leeks, asparagus and celery. As there is an involvement with oxalic acid these foods need to be monitored very carefully. Off she went home to Bridgwater with her husband, both in a very positive frame of mind, knowing that something could be done, and that she did not have to live with it. She came to see me some three weeks later, the swellings had disappeared, she was sleeping through the night and the pain was a thing of the past.

Some time later she was so busy with work, running a home, being a Mother etc; that she wandered from the straight and narrow and very quickly all the symptoms returned, she was told in no uncertain terms that she was "the boss", and if she wished to stay well the ball was very firmly in her court. I can diagnose, test, tell you all the pitfalls and put you on the right road to recovery but ultimately it rests with you. There is a saying I use with patients that I feel expresses it well - " Your body is the Church within which you worship, how you worship is entirely up to you".

YOU DO NOT HAVE TO LIVE WITH ARTHRITIS!!.

CHAPTER TWO

PESTICIDES, SPRAYS, DRUGS AND ARTHRITIS

If you know anything about modern food production you will not need me to tell you that pesticides and sprays are in constant use. I referred earlier to the pesticides and sprays being used on pastureland, nitrìtes, nitrates, growth promoters, weed killers etc. The cattle feed on this and it ends up in our meat and milk. They are usèd to spray the potato crop while growing and again when they are put down for storage.

My wife was asked a year or so ago to carry out a favour for a friend of ours,to collect the pesticides for his potato crop, she had to sign three poison forms. A patient of mine is a very large potato grower in Kent, and when I mentioned about not eating the potato skins when baked, the reply I received was, "don't be silly, we would not eat those, we have a large patch for our own consumption".

Buy **ORGANIC!!** Your apples are sprayed so often it is unbelievable, and I have yet to test a patient who does not react to apple skin. Buy **ORGANIC!!** If they are not organic then please make sure you peel them. I am beginning to sound like a one man advertising campaign for the Soil Association. They do an admirable job and you will see the Soil Association logo on foods that are acceptably organic. But that is not the reason I am mentioning these things, I am referring to clinical reactions, not just test results, but the reports I receive from patients who have ingested something unsuitable, they can be quite severe and often take as long as five days to clear the system, and as long as three weeks for balanced health to return. So beware! !

I would like to quote from a book called The Pesticide Conspiracy by Professor Robert Van Den Bosch, it is the last page. " Nature is emitting signals warning us that under the existing format the future is ominous. She is saying that that we cannot continue our attempts to ruthlessly dominate her and that if we persist disaster is in the offing. She has many voices, and of the clearest is that of the insects. The insects have already told us that we cannot overwhelm them and that there has been a price to pay in trying.

But, Nature has other voices, and if we listen carefully we can hear these additional warnings too: the voices of the trees in the crashing forests before an assault of axes, and the later rumble of a mudslide as a cloudburst sweeps the denuded mountainside, the voice of the soil in the crunch of the alkali beneath the boots of a farmer pacing his land ruined by bad irrigation; the voice of the water as it roars crystal clear through the penstocks of a mighty dam, leaving behind the nutrients that once nourished a great floodplain and fed a vast fishery; the voice of the wind as it hisses with a load of dust whipped from the topsoil of half a county. Yes, the voices of Nature are quite easy to hear - if we will only listen. The question is, will we?. And if we do, can we overcome our corrupt ways and marshall our efforts to collaborate with Nature as her brightest child and shepherd of Earth's life system?. If not, it is almost certain that things will worsen for Nature, but even more so for us. Then at a certain point in time we may no longer be able to cope with the adversity and we will perish. But Nature will survive, and so, too, will the insects, her most successful children. And as a final bit of irony, it will be the insects that polish the bones of the very last of us to fall."

This was written and published in 1978. It does not take a lot of imagination to realise how prophetic these words were. For nearly twenty years later we are seeing the natural resources of this world threatened, and the natural kingdom occupying the land and the sea being polluted to the point of extinction. Is it really surprising that fishermen patients of mine tell me that they would never touch the fish, or let their families do so, because they are so diseased through pollution. Potato growers who will not eat the produce they sell to the public, apple growers who save private orchards for their own consumption, the list is endless. Just consider the billions of pounds spent on additives and preservatives in this country alone, and you will see why there are cartels to protect them, and intentionally deprive you of the information that is rightly yours.

It really depends on you the public demanding **NATURAL** foods, uncontaminated by pesticides and sprays, additives and preservatives, and genetically engineered, or irradiated, so that those in power will listen and act upon the pressure you exert. Even politicians realise that it is the public that put them in offce, so contact your local Member of Parliament if you have a complaint.

DRUGS AND ARTHRITIS

N.S.A.I.D.S. Non Steroidal Anti - Inflammatory Drugs.

The first thing to notice is they are drugs. I have not come across one drug that does not have one or more side effect, or contra indications. Look in MIMS, Monthly Index of Medical Specialities. Have you noticed the portent of the title ?. Monthly Index- why on earth do we need a monthly index of drugs available for prescription by G.P.'s.?. I think you know as well as I do, new drugs, or old drugs under a new name are introduced every month, old drugs are taken off for one reason or another, such as Opren referred to earlier. What a blessing that it was removed before too much damage was done. As I was saying, look in MIMS and there is not one drug that does not have an addendum that states quite clearly "side effects". The most common side effect I have come across is that all NSAID's cause disturbance to the digestive system, or even stomach ache. Prolonged use of these drugs can lead to haemorrhaging, you will often find that when these drugs are prescribed you will also be given Gaviscon or Zantac or another antacid to combat the symptoms.

Another very important factor as far as I am concerned is that all NSAID's, bar one, contain lactose. I can hear you saying now "which one does not contain lactose?". I have been assured by the manufacturers that it is Voltarol Retard. Note the Retard, it is very important, ordinary Voltarol still contains lactose.

I take a monthly newsletter called" What Doctors Don't Tell You". If any of you reading this book are interested in caring for your own, or your families health, I would strongly recommend you subscribe to this magazine. I will give the address in the Useful Addresses section in the rear of this book. If you are only interested in the arthritic condition I strongly recommend you to send for the special pack which contains :- **ARTHRITIS ; THE PRICE OF PAINKILLERS and ARTHRITIS ; SECOND LINE TERRORS.**

Once you have read these you will see why I recommend that you find out from a qualified practitioner, what your allergens are, the correct diet to follow, and how to free yourself from taking drugs. I do not intend to quote continuously from these newsletters, but I cannot resist referring you to the two sub headings of the pack I have just mentioned. " **NSAID's for arthritis account for 2,600 deaths and 20,000 emergencies each year ".**

Followed by : **" Arthritis treatment seems to be a stumble in the Dark "**. Hence the title of this book, far too many people, thousands, if not millions are given the impression that all they can do is to take drugs, and learn to live with it. Not true - **Lighten Our Arthritic Darkness.** Hard hitting headlines I am sure you will agree, but it is a hard hitting disease, and the general public are not made aware of the risks they take with using these drugs. Writing in The New England Journal of Medicine.13 June,1991, the Australian rheumatologists Dr. Peter. M. Brooks and Dr. Richard. O. Day state the following:- The gastrointestinal effects of NSAID's include gastric erosion, peptic ulcer formation and pertoration,major upper gastrointestinal haemorrhage, and inflammation and change in the permeability of the intestine and lower bowel. Brooks and Day quote another study showing that the risks of being hospitalised due to the gastrointestinal adverse effects are "seven times that of patients not given NSAID's. " These results led these two investigators to suggest that in the United States the syndrome of NSAID's associated - gastropathy accounts for at least **2,600** deaths and **20,000** hospitalisations each year with patients with rheumatoid arthritis alone ".

I have to say that in all my years of treating patients who have taken NSAID's, and some of them for considerable amounts of time, none have actually died from them. I have however, had quite a few that have been hospitalised with severe haemorrhaging and quite seriously ill. Many, many others have had warning symptoms of gastro-intestinal disturbances, and have taken themselves off NSAID's. It would be fair at this point to mention that no drug cures the condition. NSAID's in particular mask the symptoms, reducing the pain level and some inflammation, but allowing the condition to rage throughout the whole system, unchecked. Think carefully about this : Is pain there for a reason ?. Of course it is. It is natures way of telling you that something is wrong with the system, there is dis - ease. The drugs mask the pain and lull you into a false sense of security.

I know the pain of arthritis, and I also know how easy it is to take drugs to give you some rest from the pain, and allow you to sleep, but do think very carefully before doing so, and if necessary go to your library and look up the drug and it's side effects.

Bearing in mind that it only masks the symptoms, it would do you, or any of your loved ones that are suffering and taking NSAID's, to check with your G. P. what the side effects are, and if there could be long lasting damage?. Remind yourselves and them

YOU DO NOT HAVE TO LIVE WITH ARTHRITIS!!

Rheumatologists are beginning to routinely prescribe an alarming range of drugs whose side effects range from death, blindness, cancer and mental disorders. Many of these drugs are powerful immunosuppressants and cell blockers.

Now, stop!! Take a deep breath, carefully read that last sentence again. Does anything strike you as odd?. I am sure you have realised that the one thing that we need to fight infection of any kind is a healthy immune system, and a healthy cell structure, yet here you are being prescribed drugs by a rheumatologist, a specialist in his field, the very thing that is going to suppress that which you should be restoring and **preserving.** Can this possibly be the route to take?. I certainly would not take it, and I certainly would not advise one of my patients to follow it, for to my mind it can only lead to disaster in the long term. I do grant however that in the short term it may offer some relief if the condition is extremely severe.

So many of these drugs now being prescribed for arthritis were never meant for this condition in the first place and are prescribed on a purely speculative basis. They might help. There are no might's, if's or but's in the course of treatment I am recommending you to follow. It is not always easy, it is not always convenient, it certainly is not the soft option but it is a SAFE one. Let us look at some of these drugs :-

METHOTREXATE

This drug in the wrong hands is a potential killer, causing liver and kidney damage, lung disease and bone marrow suppression. Physicians Desk Reference,1992, PDR, the US drugs reference bible, reports deaths among patients on the drug. It stresses that the drug should only be given by "physicians whose knowledge and experience included the use of anti-metabolite therapy'.(Substances which fundamentally change the body's metabolism). As you can see a very powerful drug. When taken with other drugs such as NSAID's they form a lethal cocktail. Methotrexate is one of a family of drugs called SAARD's, (slow acting anti-rheumatic drugs). These are considered as second line treatments. What exactly does that mean ?. It means that the first line treatments of choice have not worked effectively and something is needed to slow the condition down, and hopefully prevent further damage to the joints.

PENICILLAMINE

As the name suggests this is a component of penicillin and was developed originally to treat Wilson's disease (copper accumulation in the liver). For the arthritic condition the daily maintenance dose can be as high as 750mg, although the patient is usually started at 125mg and 250mg to test for adverse reactions. As usual there are side effects and the most common ones are :- skin rash, mouth ulcers, loss of taste, and a more serious reaction can occur where there are skin eruptions, the treatment should be stopped immediately. The blood disorder thrombocytopenia is common and can be severe, (Drugs and Therapeutic Bulletin,1993:31:18).

SULFASALAZINE

Sulfasalazine is one of the family of cytotoxic drugs which block the growth of cells. Serious side effects include bone marrow suppression, increased risk of infection, infertility, cancer and defects in the embryo, (G.W. Cannon & J.R. Ward, Arthritis and Allied Conditions, Lea & Febiger, Philidelphia,1989). The drug was originally developed to treat ulcerative colitis and Crohns disease. (ABPI Compendium Data Sheet,1993-4).

CHLOREQUINE/ HYDROXYCHLOREQUINE

These are anti-malaria drugs that, through trial and error, have been found to have some beneficial effects on rheumatoid arthritis. They were used to treat a number of conditions after the Second World War. A common side effect can be visual impairment, even leading to blindness;

the drugs may cause lesions on the eye in doses above 6mg a day (Arthritis/Rheum 1979;22:832). Other side effects include tinnitus, insomnia, hyperactivity and anaemia.

CYCLOSPORIN

This immunosuppressant, originally developed to stop the body from rejecting transplant organs, is the current flavour of the month in medicine, used to treat every disease doctors otherwise don't know how to handle. It acts by lowering the immune system T-Cells and should be used in treating rheumatoid arthritis only when the condition is life threatening.

Other immunosuppressants that may be recommended include Azathioprine and Cyclophosphamide, although they come with the same high risks. **None are licensed in the United Kingdom for the treatment of arthritis, although they are being investigated.**

Should we really be looking at suppressants of the immune system, particularly when they are only being investigated?. I think not. We should be looking for the causatory trigger of the breakdown of the immune system, and, once determined, eliminate it from the diet and allow the immune system to recover naturally, which thankfully it does, and more speedily, with some help and support.

STEROIDS

After immunosuppressants, steroids are the most controversial - and possibly the most damaging - treatments available for arthritis. Steroid overuse in the 1950's to treat arthritis and the horrors that came from that, has put paid to the treatment among those Doctors with long memories. The Medical Research Council trial in 1960 concluded that the risks outweighed the benefits .The side effects of the glucocorticoids - which include cortisol, cortisone, prednisone and dexamethasone - are many and various. These include the suppression of the immune system, osteoporosis, muscular dystrophy, peptic ulcer, psychiatric disorders, infections and eye problems (T.W.Behrens and J.S. Goodwin, Arthritis and Allied Conditions, Lea & Febiger, Philidelphia 1989).

I wish that I could agree with the above statement that most have learnt from the 1950's. I see patients every week who are on steroids, mainly Prednisone, and some have been on it for as long as five years. One only has to look at these patients and see the damage that has been done to realise how suppressing the immune system fools the body and masks the pain, while destroying kidney and liver function and causing deterioration of the bone structure, osteoporosis!!. However, I have to be honest and say that my impression is that rheumatologists are becoming less eager to put patients on steroids long term these days. Let us hope that trend continues, and perhaps one can hope that one brilliant, bright day, they may start looking for the cause, instead of looking for a drug to suppress it. It will not happen in my days in practice as those days are already gone, but, hopefully this century, and when I have correlated all the evidence from questionnaires sent out to patients, and sent them to the British Medical Association for their perusal and hopeful acceptance, the doctors and specialists will be able to do what they should be doing, and what I have been doing for all these years, help their patients to get better.

YOU DO NOT HAVE TO LIVE WITH ARTHRITIS!!!

ANTIBIOTICS

When penicillin was discovered it was thought we had a **magic bullet.** It would kill all bacteria and cure all bacterial infections. Lìfe would be so wondertul if it was as simple as that. Pop a pill and all will be well. Of course it did not work like that and unfortunately we have had the hard lesson to learn, that by using antibiotics as the cure all, the bullet has turned on us and shot us in the foot. Bacteria learn to adapt and become resistant, our former wonder drugs are now all but useless. Did you realise that antibiotics only treat bacteria. Many of the deadly infections today are caused by viruses and antibiotics are useless against them. We can be infected by fungi too, and antibiotics encourage fungal growth. Candida albicans, of which later, is one of them. Consider this point carefully please :- Every time you take an antibiotic you are giving the bacteria around you a new opportunity to develop resistance. Remember my comments about organic food - every time you eat milk, cheese, eggs and most meats, unless they are organic, you are being exposed to antibiotics. Livestock are given daily doses virtually from birth, because antibiotics are growth promoters, and keep milk and eggs fresh for much longer, thus increasing farmer's profits.

So, what is the consequence?. Fewer and fewer antibiotics are effective against deadly infections. Patients who contract serious infections like pneumonia, or pick up a hospital infection like the deadly staphylococcus often die because the bacteria are so resistant. The recent E-Coli outbreak in Scotland is a typical example. In America, New York in particular tuberculosis is becoming epidemic, and it is quoted as affecting as many as 1 in 3 of the population, and it is antibiotic resistant. Do not be complacent it is also making a comeback in this country too.

Because of antibiotic abuse we have lost the **"war".** Remember the last outbreak of Influenza in this country this winter,(1996/7), thousands of people were affected, it lingered on for months, and what were many told when they went to their GP, "well, you have influenza but there is nothing I can do for you, or give you as they do not work, so go home and it will burn itself out eventually". Now that really does give you confidence doesn't it!. Think long and hard please, there are alternative ways of approaching illness of any kind, and protecting and strengthening the immune system is one way of doing just that.

Alexander Fleming, who discovered penicillin warned nearly a century ago that overuse of antibiotics would create resistant bacteria.

ALTERNATIVES

Yes, there are some very good ones. I can remember recently attending a meeting where the general body of the public were against a road being driven across the only piece of Green Wedge left in Taunton, and a local planning offcer stood up and said, " I am sure you are right, the Green Wedge should be preserved, but do not criticise the existing plans unless you have an alternative". Well, I have certainly criticised the use of drugs for many years and thankfully I can suggest alternatives. They are certainly many and varied, and I have tried most of them over the years, on myself and my patients with varying degrees of success. However in the last three years the most effective, and therefore the most successful, are the first two mentioned. These are not drugs but natural supplements.

N.A.G. (N-Acetyl Glucosamine).

You can imagine the comments passed by husbands when I suggest the wife takes NAG. The reasons are listed below.

Tissues in and around the joints get damaged because lubricating synovial fluids in the joint spaces become thin and watery, instead of thick and elastic.

There is a loss of the natural cushioning and consequently the bones and the lining cartilage's collide and scrape together inside the joint space.

A loss of cushioning by watery bursae allows tendons to rub against the hard edges of the bones. Cartilage starts to erode and problems arise.

Glucosamine helps to restore the thick, gelatinous nature of the fluids and tissues in and around the joints, and in between the vertebrae. N Acetyl Glucosamine and Glucosamine Sulphate are among the types of biological chemicals that form hyaluronic acid, a major cushioning ingredient of the joint fluids and surrounding tissues.

Glucosamine may therefore give good results in a short period of time for the following indications:-

* **degeneration,** swelling and inflammation of the synovial fluids.
* **osteo-arthritis** during recovery of injuries, after operations and during recuperation.
* **damage** to and inflammation of the attachment muscles.
* **dystrophy** of joints associated with ageing.
* **injury** and loss of elasticity of intervertebral discs.

* **use preventively** in cases of overburdening of the joints, for example, intensive sport, poor work posture, heavy lifting, generally in ageing and so on.

I have used this product for several years now and the results in the main have been most encouraging. There has been the odd patient who reported that it appeared to upset the stomach, so it was discontinued, and there is a very good reason for this as I shall explain later. If you try any alternative supplements and they appear to cause a reaction then discontinue immediately and have a word with your practitioner. This product is available from :- Biocare Ltd. 0121433 3727, or The Nutri Centre. 0171436 5122.

B- ALIVE

This product has revolutionised the recovery of my patients in the last three years, surpassing anything I had used previously. I take two tablets daìly every day and will continue to do so ad infinitum. I recommend all my lady patients over the age of thirty five to take it to prevent osteoporosing, **not HRT,** the so called elixir of life for women in the menopause, more of which in a moment.

There is an excellent booklet called Away With Arthritis written by the man who helped to formulate the product, Dr Rex Newnham, you will find his name and address in the useful addresses section at the rear of this book. It is an excellent read and explains how the condition occurs, what B Alive does to ameliorate the condition, and how it does it. The firm that supplies B-Alive in this country, and the booklet, are Hildreth & Cocker, 0181 675 2755.

B Alive is sold under different names in various countries. In the United States it is known as Osteo Trace and is available as follows:- OHIO and surrounds from Dr

Don Brenn,1535 NLimestone St, Springfield, OH 45503. Tel: 513 3903557.

CALIFORNIA - Mumme Enterprises,1321, Meridian Ave, South Pasadena, CA 91030. Tel: 213 2554550.

NEW ZEALAND - BORE-REX are on sale at most health shops throughout the country, and BOREXON is available from many chemists. If you have any problems obtaining these products then try the wholesalers, Bore-Rex New -Zealand, PO 58-728, Greenmount, Auckland. Tel: 09 2741630.

SOUTH AFRICA

RAY-REX tablets are available at most good pharmacies, failing that from :- Jacobs Pharmacy, PO Box 2562, Durban, 4000.

Initially these boron supplements were sold under the name BoreRex, but that name was too close to other registered trade marks in some other countries, so the name had to be changed. However, these are the only boron supplement tablets that have been submitted to and passed hospital trial. They were shown to be effective with 70% of cases that completed the trial; and these were all severe cases with the average age of 64. When younger people use these products as a preventive measure we can expect nearly 100% effectiveness.

Quite rightly Rex states in his booklet " **that if people were encouraged to prevent their illness in the first place there would be no need for hospitals. Healthy people do not need hospitals".**

Quite naturally I would agree with him and after all that is what this book is all about really, the prevention of, or recovery from arthritis without the need to use drugs. I must say though, as it is with many supplements, it is " horses for courses ". Some need as many as six daily to start with then reduce down to two to three daily, whereas some patients can only cope with one daily, thank goodness we are all different. If you do have an adverse reaction, do not give up completely, leave them alone for five days, then introduce half a tablet daily for a week, then increase at a half tablet each time until you reach the recommended dosage. You should find that it works effectively.

COD LIVER OIL

I have recommended this to patients for as long as I can remember. You will also find that throughout this book I will relax into the modern idiom and abbreviate it wherever possible to CLO. There are different strengths available, the ordinary strength you are recommended to take 4-6 at night two hours after the evening meal. The High Potency One daily are to be taken 2 at night for the first three weeks, then down to one at night two hours añer the evening meal. Why is it necessary to be so pedantic as to say two hours añer the evening meal ?. For a very good reason. We try to cheat the liver!!. Because the liver is the " sponge" or the "pantry' of the body. As arthritics we need to cheat the liver and create a diversion by eating our evening meal. The liver is then busy digesting and disseminating to other organs, whilst it is busy doing this, two hours after the evening meal we take the CLO and sneak it past the liver so that it can help to build new tissues throughout the body. In so doing it delivers oil to the joint linings and cartilage to check osteo and rheumatoid arthritis. It can fill the sac with oil in bursitis, lubricate the muscles in myositis, cover the nerves with oil in neuritis, and nourish the connective tissue in fibrositis. There has been controversy recently over the toxicity of Cod Liver Oil and I can assure you that the one from Biocare is checked regularly and is safe. Biocare 0121433 3727.

EVENING PRIMROSE OIL

A report in the Lancet reveals that evening primrose oil is effective for a substantial number of patients suffering from rheumatoid arthritis and is therefore worth considering as a nutritional supplement.

There are various brands on the market and you must check to ensure that it states on the ingredients, pure evening primrose oil, no padders, fllers etc; the one that has been most effective for me is called GLA - Gamma Linolenic Acid from Biocare Ltd. 0121 433 3727. One or at the most two of these daily is usually enough to relieve the symptoms.

In recommending these products I do not wish to infer that other products on the market are not suitable. There are many, and I have tried most of them, but I have found the products I mention to be the ones that have produced the best results for me.

I mentioned earlier The Nutri Centre,7, Park Crescent, London. W1 N 3HE. This centre stocks most of the leading brands of supplements available today and I am sure a phone call to discuss the matter would be met with a helpful response and good advice.0171436 5122.

Whilst on the subject of supplements, it has become increasingly evident over the last few years that there is a definite link between arthritis and candidiasis - Candida Albicans. In simplistic terms this means an over population of candida albicans in the gut and causing a dysbiosis, an imbalance. Certainly the parasite most commonly associated with arthritis is Endolimax Nana. If treated correctly relief can be obtained quite quickly. The condition itself is a complicated one and needs expert guidance by an experienced practitioner. I have just received and read a book by Jane McWhirter called The Practical Guide to Candida. It not only explains the condition but has a list of practitioners specialising in the condition, I would advise you to consult someone on this list if you are suspicious that this may be your problem. For copies of the book please send to Green Library, 9, Rickett Street, London, SW6 1 RU. Price £7-50 plus £1-25 p&p. All proceeds from this book will go towards research on the holistic and clinical treatment of candidiasis.

When I finished this book on arthritis I had every intention of writing one on Candida Albicans. Jane, you have saved me the trouble. Both you and Gill Jacobs have covered every possible aspect of treatment for this condition and anyone suffering with candida, and reads these books will no longer feel alone. Brilliant!! I will certainly be using the book as a reference guide to encourage my patients who come from all over the world, to follow up their treatment by consulting someone in their area who is qualified to help them recover. It has long been a belief of mine that candidìasis is responsible for many of the ills we see today.

Ten years ago I saw on average four patients a year with candida, and they were all over the age of sixty. Now I see on average, five patients a day with this condition and most of them are under thirty, and far too many are young children. It is in my view, epidemic in this country, if not the world, and the sooner the medical profession as a whole realise this, the healthier we shall all be as a nation. The most recent estimate is 28 million cases in America.

While on the subject of the relationship between arthritis and candida, it is important to state the current findings. Once the arthritic diet, with the elimination of allergens has been carried out for three weeks, and there is no sign of any improvement, then obviously one starts to look for possible culprits. As it is recommended on the arthritis diet to take molasses, a pure sugar derivative, and the fruit is limitless, then, as a precaution the molasses is eliminated, along with honey, mushrooms and root vegetables, and the fruit limited to apple, pear and banana for a further three weeks to see if the condition responds.

If it does not respond then you must contact your practitioner.

He will carry out tests to see if there is a pre-disposing candidiasis and advise you which medication to take. I would certainly take a faecal sample, send it off to the laboratory and ascertain if the parasite Endolimax Nana or candida were evident. If the results are positive and medication is prescribed it is amazing how quickly the condition responds.

If you purchase the book by Jane McWhirter The Practical Guide to Candida, which I highly recommend, you will find a list of practitioners in your area who should be able to help. You will see my name and address in there at present but do bear in mind I have now retired, and am available for postal consultations only. That is one of the main reasons for writing this book. I do not feel I can just fade away into the sunset without helping all those who suffer with arthritis to have the opportunity to avail themselves of the accumulated evidence of all these years.

So, if you have arthritis, have tried the diet for at least six weeks and nothing has happened to improve the condition, do not give up, there is always a reason, find a practitioner near to you, explain what you have done, and give them a chance to correct things, you should improve within three weeks.

I referred earlier to the product B-Alive that has helped so many of my patients over the last three years, and the man responsible for this product Rex. E. Newnham Ph.D. D.O. N.D.. There is an explanatory leaflet that Hildreth & Cocker send out with B-Alive so those of you that order it will be familiarised with the product. However I think it will do no harm to put some of that leaflet information into this book, at least you will have a good flavour of what the product does.

NUTRIENTS FOR RELIEVING ARTHRITIS.

BORON is essential for all green plants and when the content of boron in the plant is down to about 1 part per million those plants fail to grow properly; apples become brown and fibrous or corky, potatoes develop hollows with brown edges, brassicas develop hollow stems and poorly formed buds. Until the 1960's no one had been able to show any need for boron in man or animal, but then it was discovered that boron would correct much arthritis, both rheumatoid arthritis (RA) and osteoarthritis (OA). The first paper announcing this was in 1979 (Newnham,R.E.," Boron Beats Arthritis ,ANZAAS, Australian Academ of Science, Canberra, 1979).Dr Forrest Nielsen of the US Human Research Centre in North Dakota in 1987 tried boron on post menopausal women. These women, on a typical institutionalised diet that contained only 0.25mg boron a day were losing calcium at the rate of 117mg a day. When they were given a boron supplement of 3mg the calcium loss dropped to ó4mg a day(Nielsen FH,Hunt CD, Mullen LM, Hunt JR,: "Effect of Dietary Boron on Mineral, Estrogen and Testosterone Sc,1987).A pilot clinical trial was started in Melbourne in 1983 and after 5 years it was completed. It was designed for OA patients only and of those that completed the trial 70% responded favourably when using boron but only 12% on placebo (Travers RL, Rennie GC,Newnham RE, "Boron and Arthritis:The Results of a Double Blind Pilot Study', J of Nutritional Medicine,1.1990). In this trial some people apparently also had RA and they opted out of the trial. RA patients invariably suffer an early aggravation or Herxheimers reaction after the first week or two, but then after another two or three weeks they normally get quite better. Even people whose hands were bent and twisted so as to be really useless, were able to sew and knit or weave after treatment with boron. Systemic lupus erythematosus is a severe form of RA and this responds just as well. Young children with Still's disease or juvenile arthritis will get quite better in just a few days.

OA patients will recover without any aggravation. OA often comes after severe damage to joints, such as found in footballers and those who drive earth moving machinery. Some respond in just a few days but generally speaking those under 60 respond in the first month, those in their 60's take 2 months, those in their 70's take 3 months and those in their 80's and 90's can take over 3 months.

We know that fluoride will give dental fluorosis when there is an unevenness in the enamel of the teeth, but this also occurs in every bone of the body as skeletal fluorosis.

People in some parts of India and Africa who have too much natural fluoride have endemic fluorosis and can hardly stand up or work. Boron is the natural antagonist to fluoride. People who drink fluoridated water will develop skeletal fluorosis, but their doctors were never taught about this and they just call it arthritis. This is corrected with boron.

Those with broken bones are advised to take a boron supplement as boron works through the parathyroid to speed up bone minerilisation. Broken bones will heal in half the normal time when boron is taken quickly after the accident. A sheep dog was run over and sustained a broken pelvis, he was not really expected to live, but he was put on boron and is now back at work, just as lively as ever. Horses have also recovered from fractures. When a person has arthritis it is wise to take 9mg a day and then reduce it to 3mg a day a month after all arthritic symptoms have gone. This is the maintenance dose to prevent recurrence of the trouble. Those with Osteoporosis are advised to take 3mg a day, after first using 3 tablets a day for 3 months.

It is wise to only use boron in a form that has been tested and proven in a proper hospital trial. Some tablets, for example, contain chelated boron and this means that the boron is tightly attached to some other organic molecule. We want the boron readily available and not tightly combined to anything.

Nielsen's work in the USA has shown that boron will naturally raise the level of hormones in the body to the normal level. (Hormone replacement therapy or HRT is used by some people to try to overcome the effects of osteoporosing, but there is risk of cancer with the therapy).

Boron is not stored in the body, so frequent small doses are required, this being more effcacíous than one larger dose. Soil that has had much chemical fertiliser tends to have less available boron so that the plant foods grown on these soils are less nutritious. A good apple grown without chemicals can have 10mg of boron, but the average commercial apple often has less than 1 mg of boron. It is our food production system that affects uptake of trace minerals and is responsible for more arthritis than 100 years ago.

Analysis has shown that bones and teeth from patients with RA contain less boron than is found in healthy people (Ward, NI "The Determination of Boron in Biological Materials by Neutron Radiation and Prompt Gamma-Ray Spectrometry '.J of Radioanalitical and Nuclear Chemistry,110.2,1987).

MAGNESITE is a natural magnesium mineral which is essential for good bone structure. It is essential for the metabolism of vitamin B6 and enters into many enzyme processes in the body. The parathyroids require magnesium for the proper control of calcium in the bones. (See Shils ME,1976 Magnesium Deficiency and Calcium Parathyroid Interelations P.23-46 in Trace Elements in Health and Disease Vol 2 Prasad and Oberleas Academic Press NY).

PYRIDOXINEVITAMIN B6 has been used to treat rheumatism as it reduces edema, joint stiffness, pain and sensory numbness, especially in the arms. (Dr. Ellis, "The Doctor's Report " , 1973).

ZINC is essential for many bodily functions, especially for the proper lining of connective tissue in cartilage, and for its regeneration (See Prasad and Oberleas as above).

SILICA or DIATOMITE contains silicon which is essential for normal growth in all animals and man. Its deficiency causes depressed growth and abnormal bone formation. It is essential for mucopolysaccharide metabolism and proper cartilage formation.(See Davis NT.1981. An Appraisal of the Newer Trace Elements P 173-174 in Trace Element Deficiency; Metabolic and Physiological Consequences. Ed. Fowden, Garton and Mills. Royal Soc. London).

VITAMIN B3 NIACIN/ is essential for cell respiration and is reported to help arthritic conditions. (Doctor Hoffer, "The Complete Book of Vitamins",1977).

PANTOTHENATEVITAMIN B5 has been used to treat rheumatism as it aids tissue repair. Rheumatoid arthritics have low blood levels of this vitamin according to Drs Barton-Wright and Elliot (Lancet, October 1963).

KELP is rich in iodine and boron; both these help to stimulate the parathyroid glands which in turn control the calcium in bones.

DEVIL'S CLAW is an African Herb that has long been recognised as useful for arthritis.

MANGANESE is essential for many enzyme processes and in proper use of many of the B Vitamins, which in turn help arthritic conditions. Muscular rheumatism is helped by manganese. Zinc and manganese work together to control the body levels of other heavy metals. It is found mainly in whole grains and green leaf vegetables.

COPPER is essential for the proper formation of haemoglobin and red blood cells. Arthritics need adequate blood to carry around the necessary minerals and other bone forming substances. Cartilage must also be repaired and blood helps here. Some elderly people tend towards anaemia so the blood must be built up in order to help them properly. Very little is needed but that small amount is necessary.

CALCIUM FLOURIDE is very sparingly soluble but it is absorbed through the intestine. When incorporated into the bones as calcium fluoroapetite it gives hardness and strength to the bone crystals. It stimulates osteoblastic activity and so helps in formation of new bone, especially after damage. Very little is needed but it certainly helps in many cases of osteoarthritis, rheumatoid arthritis, osteoporosis and ankylosing spondylitis. (See Blackmores Prescribers Reference A.8.1).

MOLYBDENUM helps to prevent dental caries which is really poor bone growth of the teeth, so other bones are likely to be similarly affected. Together with zinc it helps to counter the effects of other heavy metals. It is found in whole grains, seeds, beans, nuts and eggs.

SELENIUM is an anti-oxidant and will aid in the metabolism of Vitamin E. It is essential for the proper functioning of muscles and is a must for muscular rheumatism. It is present in garlic, whole grains, meat and eggs. Men and animals cannot live without it but we only need 200 micro grams daily. Remember many arthritics can not break down wholemeal flour.

COBALT is part of the Vitamin B12 or hydroxycobalamin. We need very little of it but it is essential for the liver and proper blood formation. It is present in meat foods, especially liver(organic only), and vegetarians are often short of this vitamin. Its presence ensures better growth and resistance to disease. Pregnancy makes big demands on the body's reserves of this vitamin because the developing foetus must get it for proper growth.

BEE POLLEN is a natural source of boron and is rich in trace elements.

EQUISETUM/HORSE TAIL is a Herb rich in silica and this helps to harden bones

COD LIVER OIL is rich in Vitamin D which is essential for good bone formation, growth and maintenance. Young people often get sufficient by exposure to sunshine, but the elderly and those living in northern climes can need a supplement. Oily fish such as herring, cod and mackerel have this vitamin in the proper natural form that does not adversely affect anyone.

A NUTRITIONAL SUPPLEMENTARY APPROACH TO THE RESTORATION OF DEGENERATED CONNECTIVE JOINT TISSUE IN OSTEOARTHRITIS AND RHEUMATOID ARTHRITIS.by Brian Hildreth T.T.C, C.H.R., C.H..F.

"Osteoarthritis is a degenerative disease and is associated with getting older. It's the wear and tear arthritis that is usually characterised by the degeneration of joint cartilage....As the cartilage and the other tissues around the joint break down the joint becomes less comfortable and more difficult to move..."

"Rheumatoid arthritis is the most crippling of all the arthritis conditions and appears to do most of its damage to the joints. Unfortunately it also damages the bodys connective tissues that support the bones and internal organs..." (Robert C Atkins M.D. " How to Treat Your Medical Condition Without Drugs "1981).

In both forms of arthritis, as simply and concisely stated in the quotations above, it is the breakdown and degeneration of the connective tissues in the joints (synovial membrane, hyaline cartilage, fibro-cartilage) without their replacement, which leads to its crippling effects. The degeneration is particularly painful and crippling when it is the fibro-cartilage which forms the intervertebral discs between the bones of the spinal vertebrae which is involved.

Osteoarthritis is a degenerative non-inflammatory disease which principally affects the synovial (freely movable) joints. As the disease progresses the articular cartilage gradually becomes thinner as its removal becomes faster than its replacement rate. As a result of this cartilaginous thinning the articular surface of the bones come in contact and consequent bone degeneration is the inevitable outcome.

Rheumatoid arthritis is an inflammatory disease which produces a variety of secondary changes in the body together with erosion of the articular cartilage of the synovial joints. There has been for some time controversy regarding the possibility of reversing this change in the cartilage and connective tissues through dietary measures. This argument also extends to osteoarthritis. However there is now a considerable body of evidence showing that, provided rigid dietary constraints are followed together with appropriate mineral and vitamin supplements, it is possible to rebuild degenerative tissue provided the treatment is maintained over a considerable time span.

THE DIETARY PROBLEM

For a dietary approach to the treatment of both forms of arthritis to be successful it must obviously supply the correct nutrients needed for connective tissue rebuilding and these nutrients must be of such a composition that the body utilises them specifically for their intended purpose.

In the past this "specificity' of nutritional requirements has proved to be a diffcult factor in devising anti-arthritis diets and many are characterised by stringent lists of foods to avoid together with dietary regimes often of a restrictive nature.

Allergic reactions to various foodstuffs are also a factor which must be taken into account and obviated from any diet, but once all considerations have been observed it is the actual dietary intake which must be able to supply the correct nutrients if it is to be effcacious from a therapeutic point of view. This is the dietary problem. Eliminating particular foodstuffs is not diffcult but replacing them with dietary elements which will achieve the best results possible is not easy.

At the heart of the problem is the major nutritional question what must an arthritic sufferer have in his or her diet which will supply exactly the right nutrients for restoration of degenerated, and degenerating, connective tissue?. There now appears to be no doubt that there is a group of essential nutrients for arthritic disease. These nutrients are similar to the essential amino acids and essential fatty acids. Without these nutrients the restoration of degenerated joint connective tissue is a virtually insurmountable problem.The nutrients required are a combination of amino-sugarcontaining polysaccharides known as mucopolysaccharides/glycosaminoglycan (GAG's).

CONNECTIVE TISSUE COMPOSITION

Until recently connective tissue and its structure has not received a great deal of attention. Fortunately this situation has changed and now a considerable amount of research has been devoted to it. It's chemical structure is far more complex than originally thought and it has been found to consist of mucopolycsaccharides (GAG's),hyaluronic acid, chondroitin sulphuric acid, chondroitin sulphate, chondroitin, and various proteins containing large amounts of the amino acid tyrosine. One of these constituents of connective tissue with an important relationship to chondroitin sulphate is collagen, the basic material of fibrous tissues which forms the ligaments which bind bones together, which forms the outer protective covering of the bone (periosteum), protects some organs such as the kidneys and the lymph nodes, and forms muscle sheaths (fascia), which extend beyond the muscle to form the tendon which attaches muscle to bone. The structure and composition of the connective tissue is functionally related to the circulatory system and the effciency of the circulation determines the transport of materials to it, and drainage of materials from it.

Among these materials carried in the blood to permeate through the connective tissue (oestrogen, androgens, thyroxine, adrenoglucocorticoids, adren-omineralcorticoids), is the all important Chondroitin sulphate (GAG's) which builds up depleted connective tissue such as cartilage and synovial membranes. At the same time further important actions appear to be initiated with the inhibition of enzymatic breakdown of the collagen together with an enhancement fibrin dissolving enzymes. GAG's/Chondroitin sulphate thus appears to be a necessary constituent of any effective dietary programme applied to the treatment of osteoarthritis and rheumatoid arthritis, and this has been borne out in practice.

Taken at a daily rate of 10g of (20% GAG's) powder/6-8 (95% GAG's) capsules per day together with a suitable diet, arthritic sufferers with a long history of the disease (one female with acute symptoms for ten years) all showed dramatic improvement within three weeks of commencing the supplementation of their diet. As an added "side effect" they all reported an increase in energy, but the main expression of improvement was increased freedom of joint movement with better mobility, including those with spinal problems. In a minority of patients there was reported increase in "normal" joint pain for a period of approximately 48 hours after commencing use of the supplement. It appears that this is due to regenerative processes occurring and increased activity in the target area. It is emphasised that this is a temporary increase in discomfort and does not occur in all suffers

Clinical trials conducted to date show that chondroitin sulphate has a definite therapeutic action and any arthritis sufferer can only benefit from its application to their diet.

As with all scientific explanations it is possible to be baffled by technical jargon. In this case I think Dr Hildreth has done well to keep it as open and plain as possible for the average person to comprehend. A couple of points I would like to expand slightly. The elimination of particular foodstuffs and their replacement. Certainly the most important factor of all in my experience is to determine the causatory trigger and the subsequent production of bradikinin. In simple terminology find the allergen, eliminate it and immediately the body will start to heal itself. However, the damage that has been done must be repaired - degeneration must be turned into regeneration and this where the use of B-Alive, GAG's and NAG have proved so invaluable to me in my practice and the successful recovery of my patients. I would like to finish this chapter on another case history, and some further information regarding Endolimax Nana. The case history first..

MR. A.F. from TORQUAY.

This man presented with arthritis and asthma, and is now perfectly well and working in what I call a hazardous profession, dry cleaning and laundering. He first noticed the pain and swelling in 1991 and put up with it for six months before visiting his GP. He was ínformed it was arthritis and could be given pain killers but did not accept. In February 1994 he consulted me and as well as the breathing problems he had pain and swelling in the knees, elbows, fngers and in his own words, " was particularly painful and could not walk up stairs without supporting myself, and I could not hold my golf clubs!!". Being a fellow golfer I know how frustrating that must have been.

Within four weeks he was free of pain, and swelling had diminished, and he has progressed favourably ever since, inhalers are a thing of the past and he is fit and well. Again in his own words " completely free of pain and tenderness".

YOU DO NOT HAVE TO LIVE WITH ARTHRITIS!!!

Now for the information on this parasite Endolimax Nana. It is known to be the major parasite which produces reactive arthritis, and in my experience it is only treatable by placing the patient on a candida diet along with the arthritic diet and treating the gut dyboiosis brought about by this parasite. The supplementation I have used to the greatest effect is as follows:-

Replete for one week. This is a powder probiotic which contains billions of healthy bacteria. It is common during the first few days to have a lot of flatulence, some patients report a little nausea, and some report a slight headache, this usually passes off after five days, and after the seven days of Replete commence:

Eradicidin 1 capsule 3 times daily after food.

HEP 194 one before breakfast and evening meal.

Vegedophilus one before breakfast and evening meal.

Obviously as I have stated before, every patient is different, but on average a period of two to three weeks on this regimen is sufficient to bring the condition under control. It is then essential to seal the gut and prevent any further incursion in to the bloodstream (Leaky Gut Syndrome).

Enteroguard for 10 days to 14 days as directed on tub.

Vegedophilus to be continued one before breakfast for at least a further month.By this time the condition should be much improved and you should be able to go back on to the arthritic diet with no problems. The above supplementation is available from Biocare or the Nutri Centre previously mentioned.

I am a Psoritic arthritic. What this means is that I suffer from psoriasis, a skin condition which in many ways resembles ringworm, and affects all parts of the body, I have had it in my ears and eyes, and pustular arthritis on the feet, and jolly painful it is too. Do not be complacent about this condition either. It is a well known and accepted fact within the medical fraternity that psoriasis and arthritis are bed fellows. One can lead to the other. So, if you have psoriasis take precautionary measures now, do not wait until arthritis strikes. Eliminate the dairy products first. If that does not work try the arthritic diet, and if that does not work try the candida procedure. It will be worth it I assure you.

YOU DO NOT HAVE TO LIVE WITH ARTHRITIS!!

CHAPTER THREE

CHAPTER THREE

DIET FOR LIFE

The title speaks for itself really. It is for life once you have discovered your base allergens. I would much prefer to call it a way of eating. There are so many occasions where patients have kept strictly to the recommended guidelines, observed the benefits with recovery to full health and freedom from pain. So, human nature being what it is we now think that as we are well we can go off the rails a bit, it will not hurt! ! Once you believe or assume that - you are in real trouble and heading for a big let down, the reaction is almost instantaneous. The temptation is always there, when the first reaction is negative, to continue in that vein, this is the first step down the slippery slope. **Please do not take that course.**

Let me try and explain the situation and why the reactions occur so quickly. As you detoxify and clear the system, the adrenal glands, sitting on top of the kidneys like two healthy walnuts, respond, and behave as they should by producing adrenaline, cortisone, and histamine, (ACH) to protect you and keep you on an even keel. When a suspect food is ingested the natural defences of the body leap into action and are able to cope. But if this is repeated too often the adrenal glands atrophy and the toxins are released into the system again. So, please do not be fooled. Remember what I said about the three stages of the General Adaptation Syndrome?

I would like to explain a typical reaction of the above scenario.

Richard is a large well built man and if anything was carrying a little too much weight. He is a member of my golf club, and while playing in a match together, he mentioned that he was considering giving up golf because it was becoming too painful. I then asked him why this should be and he told me he had been diagnosed as having arthritis. The hands were so painful it was difficult to hold the clubs, and hurt every time he hit the ball.

I told him he did not have to give up golf, but if he was willing to give up certain foods, and keep rigidly to a strict diet then he was to come and see me, this he duly did and we discovered his basic allergens and put him on the special diet. In a very short space of time the pain and swelling had disappeared, he had lost weight and felt much better.

This went on for some months until he informed me one day that the pain was back in his hands. I asked him if he had changed his diet in any way and he assured me he had not. I then asked if he had introduced anything new into his normal diet, "only honey and sheep's yoghurt." Could the sheep's yoghurt be too rich for the liver to cope with?. More likely to be the honey as we as arthritics do not cope with sugar too well I told him." I will cut them out and see what happens", he said. Three weeks later I saw Richard at the golf club and enquired how things were going, the reply was most encouraging, "fantastic thank you" he said. Needless to say I was much relieved but curious, so I asked if it was the honey - "well, not exactly he said," as you probably know I am a builder and I take two flasks of tea to work every day and I was putting six spoonfuls of sugar in each flask! !". An overload on the pancreas, initial reaction nil, adaptation for a week or two then Stage Three!

The immune system could not cope and back came the condition with vengeance.

Such a simple slip, but look at the disastrous results. It really is never worth taking risks unless you are sure it is safe. If things begin to go wrong, no matter how simple it may seem think carefully about a food or substance you may have recently introduced. I know by bitter experience that once you are free of arthritic pain, there really is no urgency to return to that again. It is a terrifying thought.

So, on we go to the diet, and as I have said before I would much prefer to call it a way of eating. It appears to me that once you start altering a patient's food intake they are on a diet, so we shall call it that. Once you have established your basic allergens then it is a matter of keeping to the regimen for at least six weeks to see whether pain and swelling diminish. If all is well, then you know that this is the way forward and apart from the occasional treat, **it is for life**. I will come to occasional treats later, and they are always better for the waiting aren't they?.

I would like to include at this point a paragraph by the great Naturopath Harry Benjamin M. D. **`By the very nature of the case, such quick and definite results as those which follow the treatment for simple rheumatism, can not be expected, natural treatment holds out the only cure - or even partial cure that exists for them in the world today. Orthodox medical treatment, by means of injection or otherwise, is worse than useless where real cure is concerned. The sufferer from arthritis, more so than any other, can afford to no longer tamper with their diet if a cure - or even partial cure - is wished for.'**

When you realise that this statement was made in one of his books more than **thirty** years ago, it makes you aware not only how profound that statement was, but just how much money has been wasted on arthritic research, which could have been spent more wisely researching the effect of food on the human system. The drug companies which fund these research projects would not like that. It would mean that anyone who had any respect for their body would not take drugs for fear of the known side effects, and then where would the drug companies be?

Listen to many general practitioners, and certainly the majority of rheumatologists, and they will tell you quite categorically that **food has nothing to do with arthritis at all.** When you challenge them and ask them what research has been carried out, they have no answer, because quite simply, no tests have ever been carried out in depth, or superficially. It is dismissed out of hand. In all his years of study a doctor is provided with approximately six hours training on nutrition and diet, and that only in recent years. You might just as well ask a car mechanic to do a hysterectomy. He would have about as much idea as the doctor has about diet and nutrition. Please do not think I am knocking doctors, in general, they do a splendid job under the incredible circumstances in which they work .

I believe I am right in saying that a doctor is allowed within the confines of the National Health Service only 3-5 minutes per patient for most consultations. This is to listen to what the patient is saying, test and diagnose, write a prescription or letter of referral, tab it into the computer "next patient please"!! How can this possibly be sufficient time to diagnose or treat a condition as serious as arthritis?

There are rules and guidelines to follow, and if you join a club, and I hope you will join those of us that are now free of the dreadful symptoms of arthritis, what do you do? You abide by the rules, or you do not bother to join. So here we go - gird up your loins - be ready for a change of eating and remember please **raw and organic is best,** lightly cooked and fresh is next best, frozen is third best and last of all tinned. Although having said that I have advised patients for years to eat fish and oily fish in particular and in most cases this has been no problem.

I am going to remind you again that the first seven to ten days of withdrawal are the worst, and the most common complaint in the first twenty four hours is a very nasty headache. Also remember we are all different so our recovery times are not going to be the same. So bear this in mind please and do not get disheartened if you are not free of pain in the first few weeks, give it at least six weeks, and then if nothing has changed consult your naturopath, homoeopath or nutritionist.

The following is a list of your **ENEMIES** and **POISONS:-**

Prepared foods and processed foods. Packaged deserts. Tinned soups. Tinned fruits. Tinned meats. Tinned vegetables. Tinned poultry. Cake. Sweets. Ice cream. Smoked fish and meats. Packaged cereals. Bakery products. Spaghetti. Pasta. Refined rice. Noodles. Pizza. Coffee. Soft drinks. Jams. Jellies. Sugar and artifcial sweeteners. Imitation dairy products. Fabricated foods, imitated, altered or semi-prepared by man. Wine. Beer. Liquor.

I know what you are going to say - what is there left to eat? The answer of course is a lot. Fresh fruit Garden fresh vegetables. Delicious fish and selected meats. Natural cheeses, eggs, nuts and natural sweeteners.

Which would be your choice? Apple pie and cream topped with severe arthritic pain and swelling.

OR!

Fresh, raw, mixed vegetable salad, including avocado pear, Icelandic prawns, parsley, Portuguese watercress, endives, enjoyed with a dash of healthy, zestful, absolutely pain free living?

If you are in pain and have arthritic swelling then I know which one you would chose. When I was in so much pain, had someone told me to go and eat grass I would have done so. You will not need much shelf space - that is where one stores tinned and packet food - foods that are designed to have a long shelf life, and preserved accordingly. Beware! ! anything that has on the label LONG LIFE! You know what that means. It has been treated and preserved to have a long life, and how on earth can that be natural or live food?

You will need refrigerator space for the `alive' foods. Heads of lettuce (organic if possible), cauliflower, calibrese, spring greens, spinach (preferably raw),sprouts, organic cabbage, parsley, asparagus, beans, leeks, onions, (remember it is best to blanch these before cooking), any food or fruit that you have grown yourself or you have fresh and organic you can freeze down. Fruit is also included in this except strawberries! They contain massive amounts of histamine and often cause deleterious reactions.

YOU CAN ELIMINATE YOUR ARTHRITIC CONDITION IF YOU HAVE THE WILL!!

If you have had extensive `gold' or steroid treatment then you may have to be much more patient, and even be prepared for the fact that it may not work for you at all. The irreversible damage done to blood platelets, and the structural damage, may well be too severe to rectify.

At one time, some years back now, if a patient booked in with an arthritic condition my Secretary was instructed to ask if they had been prescribed gold treatment, if the answer was in the affirmative I would not accept them. Then one day a couple came, and the wife had been prescribed gold, so I asked them why they had kept the appointment. Quite rightly, the husband said, "what right have you to deny my wife the chance of getting better". I have no right to do so, and my refusal was based on the fact that blood platelets had been irrevocably changed, and I did not wish them to waste their time or money." We are willing to try anythíng to get my wife better", he said, so, I agreed to test her and warned that recovery could take much longer. Were you warned that once taken they could have severe side effects? I asked. "No was the reply". It is amazing how few patients are. If you are a Doctor reading this, please tell your patients that gold and steroid treatment is the last straw and the long term effects of these are not known.

As luck would have it she recovered in approximately six weeks, with diminishment of pain and swelling, but judged overall, her recovery was nothing like as quick as a patient who had not been prescribed gold. But, needless to say from that day on I never refused a patient who had been prescribed gold, and thankfully many have improved their quality of life considerably since that time. It is worth pointing out that should the worst scenario occur and you do not feel any major benefits, it would still be worth doing to prevent any further deterioration. **Prevention is always better than cure.**

The real cause of arthritis is (my hypothesis) :

1. The inability of the digestive system to tolerate certain foods - **pancreatic malfunction.**

2. A scarcity of the nutrients that the body requires.

3. An overabundance of chemical additives used in the processing of foods, which our bodies do not need, and which indeed it can not cope with.

You are not going to take bigger and better pills to cure your arthritis - simpler and for some worse than that - you are going to give up some of your favourite foods of a lifetime - a bitter pill indeed for some! !

YOU CAN ELIMINATE ARTHRITIS IF YOU HAVE THE WILL!!

Here is a list of seventeen additives, which will in time, be proven to be harmful to the human system over a period of years.

1. BUTYLATED HYDROXYANISOLE - E 320.(BHA)
2. BUTYLATED HYDROXYTOLUENE -E 321 (BHT)
3. DISODIUM DIHYDROGEN PHOSPHATASE.
4. MONOSODIUM GLUTAMATE - SODIUM HYDROGEN L-GLUTAMATE E621.
5. CARAGEENAN - E407
6. FOOD COLOURINGS.
7. SODIUM NITRATE - E 250I251
8. SODIUM NITRITE
9. POLYSORBATE 60 - E 435.
10 POLYSORBATE 80 - E 433.
11 DI-POTASSIUM PHOSPHATE - E 340(b).
12 SORBITAN-MONOSTEARATE - E 491.

13 OXYGEN INTERCEPTOR.
14 SULPHUR DIOXIDE - E 220.
15 BENZOATE OF SODA - E 211.
16 SODIUM SILICO ALUMINATE.
17 CARAMEL - E 150.

Where possible I have added the E Numbers, which should enable you to use the Find Out Booklet available from Foresight, listed in useful addresses section in rear of book.

Now you are ready to start your treatment. Your body will love it. Your habit department will not. If you are a sufferer of **osteo** or **rheumatoid arthritis,** the seven day programme will be the hardest, yet most rewarding and important seven days of your life. There are many more case histories I could relate, but hopefully this one will give you heart and spur you on.

Mrs B.B. from "Nirvana" Weston Super Mare relates her story as follows:-

"In 1983 I began having severe pain and swelling throughout my body, also terrible mood swings - over the following three years my husband took me to three top specialists, who gave me every test imaginable to try and find out why I was so ill, also deteriorating so fast. On my last visit to a specialist I had got to the point where I was unable to work, either by being employed or working in my own home, i.e. housework etc.; and relied heavily on my husband and family who would clean and cook for me, as it would take me at least three hours to mentally and physically get started in the mornings, and some days even longer.

The pain by now was becoming intolerable and even holding a cup became a mammoth task. After the specialist had examined me - he informed me there was nothing he could do for me, I had arthritis throughout my body - every joint and my ribs, **and I would have to live with it.** (Note this typical reply! !). I was 47 at the time. On hearing this I discussed at home, my future, with my husband. I explained to him that if I had to live with the rest of my life in such severe pain and so mentally slow - that I did not wish my life to continue - as the pain increased, my skin became unbearable to touch - so even a re-assuring cuddle was out of the question. I also realised the rate this debilitating disease was moving that within a year I would be unable to walk, and would need a wheelchair.

A short while after this I was informed by two different people of a Mr Davies who lived in Taunton, he may be able to help me. By this time I was convinced there wasn't anyone who could help me, but decided to make an appointment to see him. So, in 1986 I went along for my first appointment with Mr Davies. On arrival at the surgery we found Mr & Mrs Davies extremely understanding to my condition. In spite of this both my husband and myself were very dubious as to whether he could help me.

Mr Davies began the tests explaining everything to us, but then told me, not only did I have arthritis, but I also had 20 other things wrong with me, such as mastitis, severe headaches, heartburn, eczema etc.; so, although we politely listened to Mr Davies saying," if I was to do exactly what he suggested then I would be cured in six weeks", we were just a little sceptical to say the least. (I would query this as I never say cure, but say that you should be feeling better).

On returning home neither of us were completely convinced by what we had seen or heard - especially after consulting "TOP" specialists in the past who could offer no help for my condition, and then, here was this man saying he could cure me, provided I stick by my "new way of living" diet sheet. We talked it over for many hours and then decided I had nothing to lose - so, lets try it, in the back of our minds we thought we would prove him wrong, as we could not possibly imagine how food could make me so ill.

The first three days were the most painful of my illness, and although Mr Davies warned me I would feel worse, I never expected to feel so bad, I spent most of the three days in bed - eventually I was able to get up, and slowly over the next few weeks I began to feel better, and at last able to have a full nights undisturbed sleep. After six weeks we returned for my second appointment with Mr Davies, I explained that I still had some arthritis in my thumb joints and ribs, he then checked me on all the other problems he had pointed out to me, and I found I only had three of them left. Mr Davies suggested that I kept a sample of all foods etc.; which passed through my mouth for the next two weeks and label them. This I did and at the end of two weeks I returned and Mr Davies checked out all the samples I had kept, eventually he found that my toothpaste was the culprit, as it had colouring in it. Within two weeks of finding this out my life changed, and since this time I have lived a pain free life,(unless I detract from the diet or eat a food I am allergic to),. I no longer have to rely on others to help me in any shape or form.

Within a year of my last visit to Mr Davies I started my own catering business, before seeing him I would have never had the confidence to have done this. A few years ago I had reason to consult my doctor, and mentioned to him that I had not seen him for five years, which was quite something, as when I was ill with arthritis I would see him weekly. I explained everything that happened to me during this time, but it was obvious he was not impressed - even when I pointed out that the proof was before his eyes.

It is now thirteen years since I became a victim to arthritis. I have a very full life, I am four stone lighter, skin and hair 100% better, I look and feel ten years younger, but best of all I am now **"PAIN FREE".** Family and friends have been so impressed at the new me they have also consulted Mr Davies, not only with arthritis, but eczema, asthma, hiatus hernia - with equally wonderful results, and we shall continue to recommend Mr Davies to anyone who will listen, as without any doubt whatsoever, if Mr Davies had not been recommended to me I would not be here today to tell my story.

My husband and I would like to take this opportunity to say **THANK YOU** Mr Davies for giving me back my life. We would be honoured if you would include my story in your book. Wishing you every good luck in the future. B.B. Weston Super Mare. March 1986".

(What she did not know when she wrote this letter was that I am now retired and only carry out postal consultations.)

Whilst on that subject, and this is really an update. I was not sure that postal consultations were going to be of any value, how wrong I was. I have several patients in Verbier, Switzerland, I shall call them Mr & Mrs K, they had friends in Zimbabwe, and the husband was in a very bad way with arthritis, and in his own words heading for a wheelchair fast. The knees so badly affected that all sport was out of the question. As I was treating the husband the wife asked me to treat her too, although her condition was slightly different, I sent them a detailed questionnaire which they duly returned and from that and the symptomology they presented, I was able to determine what the basic causatory triggers may be. They started the special way of eating together, and I was delighted to receive a detailed report some six weeks later - they were both free of pain and improving in general health by the day in leaps and bounds. So my misgivings about postal consultations were soon laid to rest, and I have to say many others have been treated since then with equal success, including friends of Mr & Mrs PvanH in Zimbabwe.

I really do not think I can add much to that. It portrays all the elements of everything I have endeavoured to explain to you. The first few weeks are very tough! !. You will have to grit your teeth and persevere, even at times when you feel you can not endure any more. You may have to go in to great depth about what you are ingesting if things do not follow the correct path. You **will** fnd that if you detract from the diet you **will** get a reaction. This could, and I am sure, will be, one of the best adventures of your life. To try varieties of fruit and vegetables not normally ingested. Getting to know the taste of good uncontaminated or nonprocessed food, perhaps for the first time in your life. You will be gladdened by your taste buds, for they will revel in the natural healthy taste of food. The one thought that must always be in the forefront of your mind is BE POSITIVE! !

So, gird your loins! ! Pluck up courage! ! Show what you are made of - and beat this dreaded disease for ever! !.

YOU DO NOT HAVE TO LIVE WITH ARTHRITIS IF YOU HAVE THE WILL!!

DIET AND ADVICE
for
RHEUMATISM AND ARTHRITIS

DAY ONE

Breakfast	**NONE**
Lunch	**NONE**
Dinner	**NONE**

Drink at least four 8oz glasses of water.

Do not repeat. If still in pain after seven days then start again with day 2 and continue this **until free of pain.**

DAY TWO

Breakfast	Unsweetened grape or prune juice. Ripe banana.
Lunch	Fresh lamb. Mixed green salad, oil and vinegar dressing. Bowl of fruit in season.
Dinner	Raw vegetable plate (Chinese leaves,celery, cucumber etc. Raw fruit salad (shred apples, pears, grapes, bananas etc.; NO CITRUS.

One tablespoon of cod liver oil, or five capsules, or one full strength capsule with a drink 2 hours after evening meal.

DAY THREE

Breakfast	Blended raw fruits. 4ozs goat or sheep milk or soya organic unsweetened milk.

Lunch	Fresh fillet of top fish lightly sautéed. Raw cauliflower or other raw vegetables. 4ozs goat or sheep milk.1 tablespoon of blackstrap molasses or 4 capsules.
Dinner	Roast chicken, blanched onions or leeks,mixed green salad. Sautéed potato. Fresh fruit salad.

One tablespoon of cod liver oil or five capsules, or one full strength capsule with a drink 2 hours after evening meal.

DAY FOUR

Breakfast	Prunes or prune juice. Rice dream. 4ozs goat or sheep milk.
Lunch	Grilled lamb chops lightly sautéed. Mixed green salad. Basmati rice. Fresh fruit.
Dinner	Halibut steak or other top fish steamed lightly. mixed salad. Half avocado. Fruit in season.

One tablespoon of cod liver oil or five capsules, or, one full strength capsule with a drink 2 hours after evening meal.

DAY FIVE

Breakfast	Fruit in season chopped up on puffed rice cereal, Rice dream. 4ozs goat or sheep milk.
Lunch	Half avocado, sliced tomato, watercress, cress, spring onions.4ozs goat or sheep milk.
Dinner	Roast duck or duckling, mixed green salad, Basmati rice. Fresh fruit. 4ozs goat or sheep milk.

One tablespoon of cod liver oil or five capsules, or, one full strength capsule with a drink 2 hours after evening meal.

DAY SIX

Breakfast	Puffed rice, chopped fruit, rice dream. 4ozs goat or sheep milk.
Lunch	Icelandic or Norwegian prawn salad. Cantaloupe or Ogan melon or fresh fruit.4 ozs goat or sheep milk. Dessertspoon of blackstrap molasses or 4 capsules.
Dinner	Lightly grilled lamb chop, large chefs salad including raw peas, string beans, uncooked vegetables and greens. Plums or other raw fruit in season. 4ozs goat or sheep milk.

One tablespoon of cod liver oil or 5 capsules or one full strength capsule 2 hours after evening meal.

DAY SEVEN

Breakfast	Sliced bananas. 4ozs goat or sheep milk.
Lunch	Lightly broiled fish. Carrot sticks and watercress. Grapes. 4ozs goat or sheep milk.
Dinner	Lightly sautéed turkey, chicken etc; raw vegetables mixed in blender. Honeydew melon or fruit in season(never strawberry). 4ozs goat or sheep milk.

One tablespoon of cod liver oil or 5 capsules or one full strength capsule 2 hours after evening meal.

SPECIAL INSTRUCTIONS FOR ALL SEVEN DAYS.

1. Take one B-Alive with each meal.
2. Drink only when thirsty, and then only juice of raw fresh fruit,Or juice of raw fresh vegetables,Organic whenever possible, water bottled or filtered. Goat or sheep milk will invariably be frozen, it is a full fat milk and you are advised to water this down to equal parts. 50%milk- 50%water.
3. Substitute foods according to taste or season.
4. Continue this diet until pain and swelling disappear.
5. Add one food per day from the allowable list Appendix. A.
6. If after three weeks things are not improving as well as hoped then eliminate the B-Alive for a week and observe, if no change then reintroduce. Eliminate the blackstrap molasses for a week and observe. If no

change then reintroduce. Watch carefully for any food that you may feel upsets you, or increases the pain and eliminate that for a week. You really will be required to become a detective and the rewards will accrue.

APPENDIX A

Non whey fed pork - **yes!** Eggs - **yes!** Vegetarian or goat and sheep cheese - **yes!** Remember, **do not cook or heat vegetarian cheese in any way.** Only buy hard vegetarian cheeses and not Red coloured cheeses.

You can add food after food to your permanent arthritis free life, one at a time every three days so that you can spot a possible culprit. Those of you that have only been recently affected with arthritis can add foods faster than those suffering with long term damage and must give time to allow their joints to adjust, Having said that, nobody - I repeat nobody - should ever return to the hard core troublemakers you have been warned about.

FOODS THAT MUST ALWAYS BE WATCHED CAREFULLY.

The more you avoid these items the safer you will be and the speedier will be your recovery.

1. Make sure you are free of pain, heat and swelling before introducing grains, porridge etc. Start with corn flakes, rice krispies, puffed rice and then white flour until you are absolutely sure there is no reaction, then you can introduce brown flour slowly, it can in some cases produce phytic acid and needs to be watched carefully.
2. All flour products like bread, toast, cakes(home baked with dairy free margarine), pizzas, pies, biscuits, crackers, doughnuts(contain milk), spaghetti, noodles etc. ;

Once all pain and swelling has disappeared and you are sure the white flour is acceptable with no reaction, then you can gently add these products(except pizzas and doughnuts).

3. Coffee, tea, cocoa, liquor, beer, wine, coca or Pepsi cola, carbonated and soft drinks. After the first week you can introduce a good tea, not tea bags, such as Darjeeling, Assam, Luaka.
4. Sugars, sweets, ice cream and artificial sweeteners.
5. Jellies, jams and marmalade. The exception to the rule here is if the fruit is organic and the minimum of sugar is used, then once free of pain they can be introduced slowly. Remember sugar is one of our biggest enemies.
6. Tinned or processed foods, custards, puddings and prepared mixes.
7. Frozen fruits. Unless they are organic.
8. Any food manufactured or adulterated by man, such as prepared breakfast cereals or semi-prepared ones like quick cooked oatmeal.

REMEMBER - LONG LIFE- MEANS - SHORT LIFE WITH PAIN!!!

<u>YOUR MOST VALUABLE FOODS</u>

VEGETABLES

Carrots, peas, black eyed peas, lima beans, string beans, pole beans, broad beans, corn, cucumber, marrow, courgette, cabbage, savoy cabbage, calibrese, young leaf spinach, kale, kohlrabi, beet tops, parsnips, cauliflower, turnips, egg plant, broccoli, curly kale, brussel sprouts, parsley, salsify, asparagus, onions, leek, chives, mushroom, brown rice, wild rice, lettuce, watercress, endive, beetroot.

FOWL

Free range chicken, duck, goose, pheasant, turkey, quail, pigeon.

MEATS

Now this is a tricky one with the current BSE scare, a tragedy really as it is something I believe should never have happened. It is easy as a vegetarian to pass comment and be flippant, and say don't eat meat. But an awful lot of people do eat it and enjoy it. Having given it a lot of thought my advice would be this - if you are over the age of fifty the chances are it is too late anyway so go ahead and eat beef, if you like it of course. It is the children that worry me, and if there is a genuine connection between BSE and Creutzfeld Jakob Disease then children should not be fed beef or beef products unless it is guaranteed **organic.** Lamb. Pork - **non whey fed**, organically reared.

I do not advise any more the ingestion of organ meats (offal), or using the juices from the cooked meat. Use marmite or Foodwatch gravy mix, or organic veg stock cubes from your health shop.

SEAFOOD

Bass, hake, bream, haddock - not smoked, cod, halibut, fresh salmon - preferably not pellet fed. Pollock, huss, gurnard.Turbot.

FRUIT

Apples (always peeled unless organic), pears, banana, peach, plum. kiwi fruit, melon, blackberry, blueberry, raspberry, nectarines, apricots, grape, currants.

NUTS

Chinese chestnuts, walnuts, brazils, butternuts, cashews, almonds, pecans, peanuts - not dry roasted. If you are a migraine sufferer then you are advised to check the citrus fruits individually and the nuts, as they can often be indicated. I would suggest that you become migraine free and then introduce one at a time and never more than two a week.**N.B. NOT HAZELNUTS.**

SOUPS

Split pea. lentil, lima bean, pearl barley, leek and potato, tomato, mixed fresh vegetables, etc.;

SEEDS

Sunflower, sesame, pumpkin, etc.; If you can obtain eggs that are definitely free range then so much better

CHEESES

Animal rennet free (vegetarian, **not cooked**). Pecorino, Cabrales, Manchego, Fetta, Chevres, Halumi, Eftaki, and often on your local market stalls or health food shops local goat or sheep's cheeses which are delicious.

WARNING!!!!

If you are a rheumatoid arthritic then you must not eat the following foods : - tomato, rhubarb, gooseberry, strawberry, beetroot, spinach, peppers, radish. Onion and leeks must be blanched before being put in the cooking. Boil for one minute and throw the water away. Some have to blanch the asparagus and celery too. It is always better to be safe than sorry! !

It does not necessarily mean that these are banished forever, what often happens is that the basic allergy trigger is removed and items such as the above can then be introduced in small amounts without any ill effects. However, this does not mean eating a lot of any particular item, it really is a little and not too often.

TEN COMMANDMENTS FOR ARTHRITIS FREE DINING

1. Balance your menu fairly evenly between proteins, fats and carbohydrates.
2. Eat some raw fruit or vegetable at every meal.
3. Avoid high heat cooking - it alters food structure and destroys nutrients. Frying with very low heat with a suitable oil to prevent food sticking to the pan is permissible. Micro waves are total anathema **- DO NOT TOUCH!!!**
4. Cook food as little as possible. Obviously in the winter months lightly cooked is the order of the day. Good home made soups etc.;
5. Save vegetable juices produced in cooking. Use in soups, gravy, sauces etc; or drink it.
6. Flesh and muscle meats are more suitable these days. Organ meats unless certain they are organic should be avoided if possible.
7. Favour whole natural food rather than extracts or parts of. Eat the skin or outer covering where edible, not just the inside. This does not apply to apples or potato skin as the residual pesticides and sprays are lethal to us as arthritics. Peel them unless you can be sure they are organic. Apple juice should only be Aspalls, Peakes, Prewetts, Appleford, and not in a carton either, bottles only please, they should be organic and marked as such.
8. Favour organic or natural sources of all meat and produce. The Soil Association do provide a booklet to

subscribers, this lists suppliers of organic foods throughout the country.

9. Avoid entirely all flour and flour products in the early stages. Everyone is different but at least for six weeks in most cases. Then introduce white flour first and ensure there is no reaction.

10. Thou shalt not commit adultery. Adulteration of foods we are talking about. There is a wonderful organisation called Foresight. Primarily set up many years ago as an organisation for the pre-conceptual care of women. The address will be in the useful addresses section at rear, they publish a superb little booklet called **Find Out,** this lists all the E Numbers in traffic light sequence - Red for danger, do not touch. **Amber** for caution and avoid if possible. **Green** for go, it is generally regarded as safe. If you purchase this booklet you will be staggered at the amount of chemicals, additives and preservatives with which manufacturers adulterate our food. These are not really good for anyone who cares about their health, but to us as arthritics they really are not permissible without paying a very real cost.

YOU DO NOT HAVE TO LIVE WITH ARTHRITIS!!

SAFE FOODS	AVOID
Organically reared Beef,chicken lamb,if not obtainable then grill meat or cook on trivet.	Meat juices,meat fat. Organ meats (liver, kidney etc;). Chicken skin (Animalsare injected with various drugs and this will avoid them).Meat stock

	from bones unless organic.
Cod, coley, huss, haddock, halibut, pollack, whiting, bass, bream,hake, sea trout, turbot Icelandic or North Atlantic Prawns.	Flatfish(Plaice, dabs , sole, flounder), shell fish (they feed on the sea bed which is polluted)
	Fish,skin coloured or smoked fish. Mackerell Herring, pellet fed trout.
Use organic vegetables whenever possible, chinese leaves are a safe salad alternative. Portuguese watercress **DO WASH EVERYTHING WELL!!**	Watercress(absorbs nitrites) Commercially sprayed lettuce, cucumber skin, potato . skin. Dutch imported cabbage. Red cabbage. Outer leaves of commercially grown green vegetables. Cherries unless organic. Strawberry.
Malvern water, Evian, Volvic, Buxton, Monastiere,etc	No carbonated waters

Olive oil (cold pressed virgin oil is best). Sunflower oil. Safflower oil. Ordinary plain potato crisps (not flavoured or low fat).

Please remember these are guidelines. The whole way of eating is manouverable to suit the individual, particularly if you are a working person. Days can be changed round, meals can be changed round as long as you keep to the basic tenets of the recommendations you will not go far wrong.

Microwaves

I referred earlier to not using microwaves for cooking. You the reader are bound to ask why. Recent research shows that microwave oven-cooked food suffers severe molecular damage. When eaten, it causes abnormal changes in human blood and immune systems. Not surprisingly the public has been denied details on these significant health dangers. In 1989 an announcement sponsored by Young Families, the Minnesota Extension Service of the University of Minnesota stated "although microwaves heat food quickly, they are not recommended for heating babies bottle. The bottle may seem cool to the touch, but the liquid inside may become extremely hot and could burn the baby's mouth and throat. Also the build up of steam in a closed container such as a baby's bottle could cause it to explode. Heating the bottle in a mìcrowave can cause slight changes in the milk. In infant formulas, there may be a loss of some vitamins. In expressed breast milk, some protective properties may be destroyed. Warming a bottle by holding it under a hot tap, or setting it in a bowl of hot water, then testing it on your wrist before feeding, may take a few minutes longer but is much safer".(Valentine,Acres U.S.A.1989).

You may well ask what has this to do with arthritis. It affects the immune system and as already stated an arthritic sufferer has a compromised immune system. Some years ago a young lad of thirteen was brought to me with rheumatoid arthritis, his joints were already distorted, thankfully he recovered quite well after a few months and all went well for approximately nine months, then out of the blue his condition began to worsen. His GP naturally said, it is a regression, rheumatoid arthritics often "flare" like this then it settles down again, or burns itself out. I do not agree with that, I was anxious to find the causatory trigger. So he came back and we tested all his foods, his drinking water, his toothpaste, everything. We could find nothing. So, I said to the parents and him and his sister, we must talk this through and find out what changed in the household at the time the condition worsened, after a few minutes Alistair said, "I know, it was when we bought the microwave". Needless to say Mum and Dad agreed this was the case and the microwave was removed from the house and his condition improved immediately.

YOU DO NOT HAVE TO LIVE WITH ARTHRITIS ! !

CHAPTER FOUR

CHAPTER FOUR

THINGS TO REMEMBER

Make sure you refrigerate oils once they are opened.

Do not re-heat oils. Use once and dispose of it.

Avoid freezing ready cooked meals then re-heating them.

Avoid re-heating meals of any kind.

Fry or roast food with oils rather than margarine. Reserve these for cakes and pastries and eat them cold.

Avoid micro-waved food entirely. It alters blood platelets within 15 minutes of ingestion whether it be cooked, thawed or refrigerated.

Use Non-Fluoride toothpaste. Boots have a very good one. There are also herbal toothpaste's without fluoride available in most Health Shops.

Avoid pasteurised goat or sheep milks where possible. The body does not cope easily with the altered state of the milk.

Avoid aluminium cookware if possible. Better to use stainless steel, glass, or enamel cookware.

Avoid overcooking food, carbon particles are deleterious.

You may well think I am being a bit over the top, but I am only too aware of the problems we have had over the years, and these are the things that have given the most cause for concern. Because, as arthritics our immune systems are under threat and our reactions to toxins are heightened. Therefore it is prudent to be over cautious rather than under cautious.

JOINT REPAIR

I have heard it said hundreds of times by patients, "once the joints are damaged there is nothing that can be done about it".

This just is not true. If it were true, the left hip I was told would need replacing by the time I was forty, would now have a prosthesis, it has not. In fact the x-rays show clearly that my hip is in a normal condition for a man of my age. I have in my possession many x-rays of patients before and after, and bone scans too, and they all show regeneration of bone after approximately twelve to eighteen months.

It is perfectly true to say that if no remedial steps are taken then regeneration of bone can not take place. But we are talking about the people who take remedial steps and the advised supplementation, then, and only then, can regeneration take place. **It really is up to you.**

EXERCISE

This is another contentious area. There are those who recommend exercise and those who are vehemently against it. My experience is that with most things, moderation is the keyword. By sitting around you are allowing calcification to take place and ligamenture and musculature to atrophy. Having said that you are then in a situation that if you do move around it is painful. It is therefore common sense to reach the halfway house, some exercise, some pain, but do not exercise to the point where inflammation takes place.

Pain is natures way of telling you something is not right, and the sensible thing to do is listen to her. I recommend that for the first three weeks whilst the body is learning to adapt to its new way of living, and inflammation is going down - do not exercise. Once you are aware of easement of pain and inflammation, and the correlation I draw here is, you were unable to get out of bed in the morning without being incredibly stiff,and the movements very limited, then one morning you wake up, swing the legs out of bed and proceed to the bathroom without pain and stiffness, then it is time to think about gentle exercise.

After all, what you are trying to achieve slowly but surely is a return to normality, but you must learn to walk before you can run. Some years ago I thought I was better, so off I went to the golf course thinking I was going to play a around of golf, after three holes I was very glad to come home again. Another case comes to mind, a patient I had seen three months previously, who had made excellent progress in that time, presented with swollen hands and wrists and fingers like little puffed up sausages. I asked the obvious question, "have you deviated from the diet?", and the answer was, "no, the only thing I have done out of the ordinary was two days ago I was feeling so much better that I pruned a few roses". I then asked, as this should not have caused that much swelling, " how many roses did you prune?". The answer she gave solved the problem immediately, "Oh! I suppose there must be forty eight rose bushes". Had she pruned four there is every chance that the hands would have remained normal.

Bones repair very easily, ligaments, tendons, and muscles take a lot longer, and it is these that you have to gently encourage back to normal usage. It is more than likely that if there has been distortion of joints then repair will take time. One of the gentlest and painless ways of recovery is hydrotherapy - swimming. Having the support of the water is advantageous but it also slows movements down and prevents damage. When sitting in the evenings watching television a good exercise for the hands is a medium tension squash ball squeezed gently but firmly for a dozen times each hand, left for an hour or two and repeated. Again, in moderation please. Do not overdo it, and the temptation is always there, if the hands are very sore next day - then you have exceeded your own capabilities - cut back! !

A good exercise if the feet are affected, is to get the old fashioned toilet roll holder with a wooden centre, take this out and when sitting in the evenings roll this under the ball of the foot, backwards and forwards in a gentle rocking movement. Same thing applies if very sore next day - cut back! !

As the condition improves and walking is possible, then this is a wonderful gentle form of exercise too. Always start on level ground and make it a short walk to start with and gradually build up. The one thing not to do if the knees are affected is knee bends. You must lie on your back, bend the legs and grasping hold of the ankles, gently pull them toward you, release, do this three or four times to start with and gradually build up.

If any of you have suffered from Halix Rigidus - the big toe becomes very stiff and a bunion starts to form - then you must gently but firmly exercise that joint by pulling the toe downwards and upwards, you may well hear grinding noises but this is nothing to worry about, as each day moves on you will find movement is increased and walking more comfortable. A gentle pull and push in the lateral plane is also of value. As the joint eases you will be able to rotate the toe quite easily.

If you have a knee problem, and in some patients both knees are severely swollen, then it is possible that after the first fortnight to three weeks the swelling will go down and the pain will ease, then some days later the pain returns. This inevitably means that the calcus formation has been broken down but the cartilage, tendons and musculature are learning to adapt to their new environment, and, being used more than normal, inflame. Ice packs wrapped in a tea towel and applied for ten to fifteen minutes twice daily often help this condition. Should the condition persist, then have an x-ray and you and your practitioner will know what to do for the best.

CONSTIPATION

It really is quite amazing how many patients report this as a life long problem. Some actually report that it is common for them to only go once a week. I need not tell you that this is not normal, and certainly will not be allowable. It is essential, as far as I am concerned that you pass a motion at least once daily. Preferably twice.

One thing I would not wish you to do is to take Senokot or any other purgative. There are various aids to help with this problem. The one that seems to suit everybody is Linusit Gold from your local health shop. Herbilax is another. The most natural way is with Magnesium Ascorbate - Vitamin C. This is in capsule or powder form and is available from Biocare Ltd 0121433 3727. This can be taken without any side effects until the stool is loose, if it turns to diarrhoea then cut back slightly. You may well find that after being on the Arthritic way of eating for three weeks the bowel settles down and no problems are encountered.

Should the problem continue then consult your practitioner, there are tests that can be carried out to ascertain the problem.

WHEN CAN I? The question that arises with every patient, and it is a diffcult one to answer.

When can I introduce bread? This, inevitably, is the first question ever asked, and the most diffcult one to answer. There are varying opinions on why the grains have such an effect on our systems, from the build up of residual pesticides which remain in the endosperm even after grading, and the fact that many arthritics can not tolerate and break down the husk and the bran in wholewheat flour and produce Phytic acid. This then produces stiffness and pain. So, the answer really is very much a trial situation. I suggest the following to my patients. Introduce white bread and see if there is a reaction after a week or two. Thankfully the numerous additives and preservatives in white flour have now been removed, but I must stress at this point that I am referring to plain white flour, many self raising flours have various reactive agents in them.

If all is well, and you are free of pain, then, and only then, introduce the whole grains, whole-wheat, porridge, barley etc.; If you notice an increase in swelling, inflammation or pain, then stop immediately. It is far better to alternate for a few weeks until the system acclimatises and learns to cope. It is never a good idea to have anything on a daily basis.

When can I introduce coffee? The answer is simple really. Never. The reactions that take place when coffee is drunk should be enough to put anyone off, and the comments usually passed are that the after effects were not worth the ingestion.

When can I introduce alcohol? The answer here is as straight forward as for grain, when free of pain and swelling. When you are sure that you are well on the road to recovery, then, as with the grains, introduce very gently and observe very carefully for any niggles or fleeting pains occurring, or even swelling. If you are clear then you are certainly advised to have real ales, brewed correctly without the use of chemicals. Guinness is an example. If you have a dairy intolerance then you would not go for a milk stout such as Mackesons, or Baileys cream, sherry etc.; Good quality white wine above Kabinett level, the price should tell you whether it is good or not. Chateau bottled red wines are worth trying but do make sure there are no reactions. Gin but not the tonic. Whisky of good quality. Vodka, but if you are rheumatoid not the Bloody Mary. I must stress because it is so important, no matter how much you may like it, you must not commence alcohol until you are positive of real improvement, and watch very carefully for adverse reactions. The biggest problem with alcohol is inding the appropriate mixer, such as tonic water, which like most of them has chemicals and additives in them which are best avoided. Soda water is alright, so whisky and soda is fine, but gin and soda? not really. Several patients have told me they water down their drinks with water quite successfully, including wine. It really is a matter of trial and error, and I would say the report back situation regarding the intake of alcohol is 50-50. So take care - proceed cautiously and ensure that you are not kidding yourself, in cheating you only cheat one person - yourself!!.

ARTHRITIS & CANDIDA

Talking about alcohol is a good lead in to warning you about the link between arthritis and candida. First of all what is Candida? In the simplest of terms it is a proliferation of yeast in the gut which has created an acidlalkaline imbalance. The candida albicans being the stronger takes over and eliminates the healthy bacteria. Because of the imbalance the mucosal lining of the gut is depleted and becomes permeable, the mycellae then enter into the blood and lymphatic system becoming - Systemic. Because it is an umbrella term it is diffcult to determine which of the protosoa, nemetodes or trophosoites is responsible. Certainly the most common where arthritis is concerned has been Endolimax Nanawhich can cause reactive arthritis. If treated properly this can be eradicated but needs to be under the guidance of a qualified practitioner.

Is there a way of recognising the symptoms of Candida?

There are several. An abnormally bloated stomach is one certain symptom. General feeling of bloat is another. Thrush in the mouth or vagina. Athletes foot. Anal irritation. Sudden onset of moles or warts. These are the most obvious symptoms to watch out for but there are others which under normal circumstances you would not associate with candidiasis. Depression, irritability, anxiety neuroses, allergies, fatigue, PMT, menstrual problems, asthma, cravings for sugar, bread, alcohol, joint swellings and arthritis. It is the opinion of many of the medical profession, that if you do not have oral or vaginal thrush you do not have candida. I would disagree with this totally. My experience over the last twenty years is that any of the above symptoms can be a pointer to the condition and should not be ignored. To ignore these symptoms is to allow a pre-disposing condition to remain a causatory factor, thereby lessening the chances of a full or even partial recovery.

The secret of finding the cause of arthritis is to follow the logical steps I have written down for you. If in doubt contact your practitioner. As a last resort you can write to me at the address shown in the useful addresses, please send stamped addressed envelope requesting a questionnaire and charges. With regard to the candidiasis then read Jane McWhirters book I have mentioned earlier, and mentioned in the books section, this will help enormously.

Today is the 28th August,1996 and the day I retire from full practice, I have seen my last patient, I might add, with very mixed feelings, but on to pastures new. Writing, teaching and training other practitioners, postal consultations, and some golf and bowls hopefully. But today, which I feel is very appropriate I received the following letter from Mrs S of Torquay.

Dear Mr Davies,

Thank you for your letter and the questionnaire on arthritis which I have answered as best I can - I hope it will assist you in writing your book - of course I have no objection at all in my name being used - I cannot sing your praises enough, you know that, how anybody medical or otherwise can dispute what you have done for arthritics is beyond me - I can only say they have never suffered the pain or they would change their minds - it is so absurd - I for one am the living proof of the wonder of allergens and the exclusion diet - and it doesn't cost expensive treatments or the threat of hip replacements and the horror of surgery.

I must admit that I came to you doubting - as I have little tíme for general medicine - being a trained nurse of the old school makes me that way - my sister Gillian made the appointment for me to see you as she was upset to see me as I was, and what a difference you have made to my life and I am sure hundreds more, may your good work carry on through your books.

I wonder if you are retiring this month as you said you were when I last saw you - I shall miss you very much even if I don't need to see you professionally it was a comfort to know you were not far away.

If I can be of any further help to you please let me know meanwhile the very best of luck to you and your wife, and may you write a best seller and make a fortune.

Best wishes to you both.

Margaret S. Devon. 22nd August,1996.

Funny really, I shall miss my patients so much, and new challenges await, but two patients have said today, we shall miss you being there as a crutch. I have never been called that before, but I think I know what they mean, it is always a comfort to know your practitioner who you have known and trusted for years, is there when you need a shoulder to cry on, or a helping hand when in trouble, and as one of my patients kindly described me, the rock. If I have been that, then I am pleased and grateful, and be assured I have not disappeared off the face of the earth, I am still contactable by post, but don't forget the sae. To all of you who read this book, I thank you for reading it, and I thank, from the bottom of my heart my patients - who have encouraged me and made me so determined to tell you :-

YOU DO NOT HAVE TO LIVE WITH ARTHRITIS!!!

Vis Medicatrix Naturae - Hippocrates.(The healing power of Nature).

USEFUL ADDRESSES

BIOCARE LTD
LAKESIDE
18O,LIFFORD LANE
KINGS NORTON
BIRMINGHAM
B303NT
01214333727

HILDRETH & COCKER
FREEPOST
LONDON
5W12 OBR
01816752755

THE PRACTICAL GUIDE
TO CANDIDA
GREEN LIBRARY
6,RICKETT STREET
LONDON
SW61 RU

AWAY WITH ARTHRITIS
REX E.NEWNHAM
CRACOE HOUSE COTTAGE
CRACOE
SKIPTON
NORTH YORKSHIRE
BD236LB

JO HAMPTON
CANDIDA COOKBOOK
46,WAINFIELD RD
SKEGNESS
LINCS PE253QT
(Practitioner specialising in Natural therapies and Candida).

NUTRI CENTRE
7,PARK CRESCENT
LONDON
W1N
01714365122

DENNIS BATES
SELECT MEAT CO
BATH PLACE
TAUNTON
SOMERSET
01823286606

KIERON & ANNE McGRATH
THE BELL & BIRDTABLE
RUNNINGTON
WELLINGTON
SOMERSET
01823663080

GWYNNE H.DAVIES
CLINICAL ECOLOGIST
4,CALWAY ROAD
TAUNTON
SOMERSET
TA1 3EQ

FORESIGHT
28,THE PADDOCK
GODALMING
SURREY
GU71XD

WDDTY
4, WALLACE ROAD
LONDON
N12PG
0171354 4592

FOODWATCH
NATU RAL PATH
CORPORATION STREET
TAUNTON
SOMERSET
01823 325022
(SUPPLIERS OF ALLERGY FOODS).

CIRRUS ASSOCIATES
FOOD AND ENVIRONMENTAL
CONSULTANCY
LITTLE HINTOCK
KINGTON MAGNA
GILLINGHAM
DORSET SP8 5EW
01747 838165

Case History -1

In October 1993 my arthritis started in my neck, I thought at the time that I had been sitting in a draught, but it did not go away. It then went to my feet with pains in my toes making it difficult to walk. At this time I went to see as Doctor, but I was told it would have to get worse before he could do anything for me.

It was about February 1994 that I first heard of Mr Davies and I then made an appointment to see him on 2nd May,1994 to fnd out what I was allergic to and also some medication, from then on I gradually improved.

At the very early stages of my treatment one of the things I was told not to eat was the jelly gravy from the chicken. I really could not understand that if I could eat the chicken why could I not eat the gravy, then one day it really got the better of me so I tried some much to my cost. I suffered for five days, so, never again!. I realised then I would stick to my diet whatever it was, and it turned out to be very strict indeed with not much choice, but I made up my mind and I really did follow Mr Davies's diet that I was advised to.

My feet were the first to get better with no pains, but my hands have been the worst to improve, I am sure I must have caused Mr Davies a few headaches, but eventually they are getting better with the exception of the fingers on my right hand which I have a bit of a job to grip things with but with Mr Davies's help I will be fine.

I feel so much better and now although in my later years, I can still bowl indoors for my County which I am sure I would never have been able to.

2nd October,1995.

Mrs A. M..H. , Minehead , Somerset

CASE HISTORY 2

Mrs D.S.
Catherington
Waterlooville
Hants

Before I consulted Gwynne Davies my condition had deteriorated a great deal since first visiting my G.P. and a Rheumatologist who could offer no hope of an improvement, and would prescribe stronger drugs. I was sent to the local hand clinic of the local hospital, who gave me hand splints to help straighten my fngers. I had reached a stage where I could not hold a newspaper without a lot of pain in my hands and forearms. I could not lift a packet of sugar, a kettle or make the beds because I could not bear the weight on my hands. I found it impossible to tum the ignition key of the car, and was so tired I needed a rest every afternoon which was totally out of character. I seldom could take a bath because I could not get out, neither my knees or my wrists were strong enough to lift me, and I could only walk a very short distance.

Within a few days of starting the treatment recommended by Gwynne Davies I lost most of the pain, and within two weeks there was a marked improvement in my health. At the beginning I weighed about 11 stone 10 ozs I am now 10 stone. After twenty one months I am a different person, much more active both physically and mentally, and I play an active part in the community again. I can now run a home, drive a car and take my dog and grandchildren for long walks. I have taken up swimming for the first time, and as a keen horsewoman I am considering riding again. It has been a wonderful cure, and every day I give thanks for the skill of Gwynne Davies. 8-10-95

Case History - 3

Miss R.D.
Chard
Somerset

Little did I imagine that the early part of 1981 would herald for me an experience which directed my journey in life on a totally new path. For several years I had been coping with arthritis which mainly affected my right knee and hands. Pain and stiffness increased and I consulted my G.P. who prescribed Opren (which constipated me), and arranged for an appointment with an Orthopaedic surgeon.

As months progressed, I needed a walking stick to get about and my fingers were so painful and swollen that simple actions like buttoning a blouse, holding a pen to write, turning a handle, gripping the steering wheel on my car, all proved intensely uncomfortable and often tears of frustration overcame me.

The Consultant Surgeon assured me that in due course I would qualify for a knee replacement!. Upon hearing this, my innermost being soared into a determined "you are not replacing anything of mine". Months passed and I felt worse, plus feeling aged, immobile and doomed.

One day a friend suggested that I consult Mr Davies in Taunton. Mid March 1981, my consultation with Mr Davies took place. After some detailed testing for foods which were likely to aggravate my condition, I was advised to eliminate from my diet foods like - dairy products, stimulants such as coffee, tea, chocolate, alcohol, acid forming foods like tomato, rhubarb, strawberries, oranges, additives, flavourings and colourings and above all wheat flour.

I shall never forget that after advising me about my diet and what supplements to take Mr Davies stated "you do not have to live with arthritis for the rest of your life; but there is nothing more I can do for you". I felt shocked and shattered - my hopes for relief from pain annihilated. Then Mr Davies added "YOU have to do it yourself'. Earnestly I embarked on my diet and in a few weeks, I felt much worse. Colleagues at work urged me to " get off that crazy diet", I felt very disheartened but was determined to persevere.

After three weeks with no improvement, I phoned Mr Davies and explained how I felt. To my astonishment Mr Davies said - " Yes, that all sounds very good to me, it is the toxins leaving your system - please persevere.". And so I did. Another three and a half weeks later after my floor exercises to ease my stiffness, I realised that I got up from the floor with new found mobility, which allowed me to bend my knees and move my hands freely. I wanted to run around the neighbourhood shouting, "Look at me, I can move and run". I was elated and phoned Mr Davies to give him my good news.

Sharing one's euphoria can be all the more poignant, especially when an individual wills the triumph over the odds for another. Mr Davies was just such a person for me.

I know that my diet is a lifetime commitment, but the benefits of mobility, good health and vitality are rewards in themselves.These qualities have enhanced my whole being, physically, mentally, spiritually and contributed to my change of career into Complementary Therapies.Rare Blessings do happen on life's journey and I shall always give thanks for Mr Davies's intervention in my healing process. R.D. 09-10-1995

CASE HISTORY 4

Mrs J.P.L.
Backwell
Bristol

Gradually I noticed my fingers were swollen at times and then they became painful. As it was during the winter of 1991/2 I was not unduly surprised. Then walking became painful - my knees ached and it was a struggle to walk our elderly dog and for me to use the motor mower to cut the lawns. I avoided bending down when possible. My hands became so akward that I had difficulty in doing up buttons, using the controls for the washing machine and the dishwasher, unscrewing bottle caps and threading a needle with sewing cotton. I had difficulty in driving my car because of the pain in my knees and inability to turn my head sufficiently to see through the rear window when reversing. At times writing was difficult and painful. I was tired and everything seemed and effort. I found that the pain in my hands kept me awake in the early hours of the morning and I could not get comfortable. Being on a diet to prevent sinusitis (recommended by Gwynne Davies), I was not keen to take any pain killers. I was warned about the future for my family and myself - fearing that I would lose the ability to do things for them and myself.

Someone suggested that I had arthritis and recommended that I took cod liver oil. I did this but the arthritis was so painful that I decided to seek medical help and visited my G.P. in February 1992. My doctor looked at my swollen hands, noticed the lack of mobility and listened to my complaint of pain - especially in the early hours of the morning. A blood test was taken and the result indicated that I was suffering from osteo-arhtritis.

In March 1992 I visited Gwynne Davies who diagnosed candida albicans as a contributory factor to the osteo-arthritis. He prescribed a diet to combat the candida albicans and arthritis together with courses of varying lengths of time of calcium caprylate (Mycopryl), magnesium ascorbate, Uritol, (Sulphur and Aesculus to overcome which I had for a comparatively short time), Bioacidophilus (changed to Vegedophilus), B-Alive, NAG (N-Acetyl Glucosamine), and Eradicidin. I now take one Multi-Vtamin tablet - cont;one Vegedophilus capsule, three B-Alive tablets, and three NAG and six cod liver oil capsules.

I have not taken any pain killers nor any anti-biotic tablets since seeing Gwynne Davies about my sinusitis in December 1989 (nearly six years).

Apart from a bad reaction one day which I think was due to die back of candida albicans and a spell of constipation, I have enjoyed excellent health. I have fewer colds than before, no sinusitis, athletes foot is a thing of the past, sore throats are minimal, scratches and cuts heal quickly and without festering, mouth ulcers (which used to be a problem) are rare, soreness inside my mouth and nostrils has gone and I am fitter than I have ever been. Having a sugar free diet has resulted in only one small filling in a tooth in six years. My little fingers have enlarged joints and only hurt when I bend them severely. Otherwise, I lead an active life and can do anything that I want to do, eg; gardening, sewing, walking, and writing without any difficulty. I am free of pain! ! Only very occasionally I get a little stiffness but it soon wears off.

For a while I was warned by the grinding of some of my joints, eg; in my neck when turning my head and in my knees when walking upstairs. NAG and B-Alive have probably helped here. Since increasing the dosage, the problem has reduced so that I am rarely aware of it now.

When my arthritis was bad, I did not think it would be possible to ever have another dog in the future. After Gwynne Davies's treatment and the resulting improvement in my health, my husband and I bought a border collie pup in July 1992. She is now fully grown with boundless energy and we walk miles together over varied terrains in all weathers. I take her to agility classes and run around the course with her without any difficulty.

At 59 years of age as a private tutor and Parish Councillor, I lead a full and active life. It involves among other things taking on responsibilities, making and keeping appointments together with resolving problems caused by other people. I find that stress makes me want to eat and I probably have too many snacks. Sometimes my hands are a little swollen and I consider that to be stress related. I keep strictly to the diet recommended by Gwynne Davies.

Having suffered arthritis, I appreciate now being able to do all the things again that were once taken for granted. This has probably resulted in cramming too much into each day without taking time for relaxation.

I am most grateful to Gwynne Davies for all his advice and help which has resulted in restoring me to good health.

J. PATRICIA LLOYD.
Mrs J. P. Lloyd, B.Sc., PGCE.
19-10-1995.

CASE HISTORY 6

I first developed arthritis in January 1986, it happened overnight. When I woke up my ankles were so sore I could not put my feet to the ground, there was no warning at all. It then spread to hands, I could not push forward at all or even turn a door knob, I had no strength in my hands in my hands at all. The arthritis in my hands crystallised and and cut the tendons in the right hand, three fmgers curled up and I needed an operation to correct it. Not long afterwards I had an operation on the left hand also. In September 1991 I spent two weeks in hospital with internal bleeding due to taking anti-inflammatory drugs. My life was very restricted and painful. I had trouble getting out of bed in the mornings, also dressing myself, my wife had to help me in and out of the bath.

I was referred to Gwynne Davies who tested me for allergies and put me on a diet, so long as I stay on my diet I can live an 80% pain free life with the exception of my elbows, these are still very painful, sad to say the joints are too badly damaged for the diet to help.

J. S. W
Kent
20-12-95

CASE HISTORY 7.

In 1983 I began having severe pains and swelling throughout my body, also terrible mood swings - over the following three years my husband took me to three top specialists, who gave me every test imaginable to try and find out why I was so ill, also deteriorating so fast. On my last visit to a specialist I had got to the point where I was unable to work, either by being employed or working in my own home, i.e. housework etc; and relied heavily on my husband and family who would clean and cook for me, as it would take me at least three hours to mentally and physically get started in the mornings and some days even longer. The pain by now was becoming intolerable and even holding a cup of tea became a mammoth task.

After the specialist had examined me - he informed me, I had arthritis throughout my body - every joint and my ribs, and I would have to live with it. I was 47 at the time. On hearing this I discussed at home, my future, with my husband. I explained to him that if I had to live the rest of my life in such severe pain and also so mentally slow - then I din not wish my life to continue - as the pain increased, my skin became unbearable to touch - so even a reassuring cuddle was out of the question. I also realised that the rate this debilitating disease was moving that within a year I would be unable to walk, and would need a wheelchair. A short while after this I was informed by two different people of a Mr Davies living in Taunton, who may be able to help me. By this time I was convinced there wasn't anyone who could help me, but I decided to make an appointmentr to see him.

So, in 1986 I went along for my first appointment with Mr Davies. On arrival at the surgery we found Mr & Mrs

Davies extremely understanding to my condition. In spite of this, both my husband and myself were very dubious as to whether he could help me. Mr Davies began the tests, explaining everything to us, but then told me, not only did I have arthritis but I had 20 other things wrong with me, such as mastitis, severe headaches, heartburn, eczema etc; so, although we politely listened to Mr Davies saying - if I was to do exactly what he suggested then I would be cured in six weeks, we were just a little sceptical to say the least. On returning home neither of us were completely convinced by what we had seen or heard - especially after consulting TOP specialists in the past who could offer no help for my condition and then, here was this man, saying he could cure me providing I stuck to my new way of living diet sheet. We talked about it for many hours. We then decided I had nothing to lose - so, lets try it! ! - in the back of our minds we thought we would prove him wrong,as we could not imagine how food could make me so ill.

The first three days were the most painful of my illness, and although Mr Davies warned me I would feel worse, I never expected to feel so bad. I spent most of the three days in bed - eventually I was able to get up, and slowly over the next few weeks I began to feel better, and, at least able to have a full nights undisturbed sleep. After six weeks we returned for my second appointment with Mr Davies, I explained I still had some arthritis in my thumb joints and my ribs, he then checked me on all the other problems he had pointed out to me, and I found I only had three of the other problems left - Mr Davies suggested I kept a sample of all food etc; which passed through my mouth for the next two weeks and label them. This I did, and at the end of the two weeks I returned and Mr Davies checked out all the samples I had kept, eventually he found that my toothpaste, which was Sensodyne - was the culprit, as it had colouring in it. Within two weeks of finding this out my life changed, and since this time I have lived a pain free life **(unless I detract from the diet or eat a food I am allergic to).**

I no longer have to rely on others to help me in any shape or form. Within a year of my last visit to Mr Davies I started my own catering business, before seeing him I would never have had the confidence to have done this.

A few years ago I had reason to consult my Doctor, and mentioned to him that I had not seen him for five years, which was quite something, as when I was ill with arthritis I would see him weekly. I explained everything that had happened to me during that time, but it was obvious he was not impressed - even when I pointed out that the proof was before his eyes.

It is now thirteen years since I became a victim to arthritis. I have a very full life, I am four stone lighter, skin and hair are 100% better, look and feel ten years younger.

But best of all I am now **PAIN FREE!!.** Family and friends have been so impressed at the new me they have also consulted Mr Davies, not only for arthritis, but eczema, asthma, hiatus hernia - with equally wonderful results, and we shall continue to recommend Mr Davies to anyone who will listen. Without any doubt whatsoever if Mr Davies had not been recommended to me I wouldn't be here today to tell my story.

My husband and I would like to take this opportunity to say **THANK YOU** Mr Davies for giving me back my life. We would be honoured if you would include my story in your book. Wishing you all good luck in the future.

Barbara Boardman
Sandbay
Weston Super Mare

OSTEOPOROSIS
The Silent Killer

Osteoporosis is the silent thief that robs your skeleton of up to 25 % of its bone mass by the time you reach 50. Osteoporosis is now a serious epidemic in Britain. This is dated 1996 so very much today. Every three minutes someone in the UK has a fracture due to osteoporosis. 1 in 3 women and 1 in 2 men have a fracture by the time they are 70 years of age. Thousands of women in their 50's suffer painful deforming fractures. £750 million each year is spent dealing with the problem. Nearly one third of orthopaedic beds are flled by patients with the condition. It is estimated that there could be 5 million sufferers by the turn of the century unless major action is taken now!!

The question is "what action do you take"?.

The old adage that prevention is better than cure must surely be correct in this case. Understanding the condition also helps you to approach the condition sensibly.

Osteoporosis is when bones become porous, and women are more at risk than men. Instead of the periosteum being like the surface of an ice rink, it becomes like blotting paper, due to the progressive loss of minerals, mass and density which can result in fractures of the hip, shoulder, ribs, vertebrae, ankle and wrist. Ankle and wrist fractures are common in young middle aged women often after a minor bump or fall. Vertebral fractures are common when over 50 and are very debilitating and painful. Hip fractures ruin 60,000 lives each year, contributing to 15,000 deaths and severe pain.

Women are more at risk than men for developing osteoporosis. The female hormones oestrogen and progesterone are protective to womens bones, just as the male hormone testosterone is protective to mens bones. So why are women at more risk than men?. From the age of 35 onwards women regularly fail to ovulate which leads to minimal production of progesterone, the major hormone for bones. Women at most risk are those who have an early menopause before the age of 45 either naturally ,or surgically by removing the womb and one or both ovaries, or those who have been on hormone treatment. Another high risk category are those women who have suffered with anorexia or bulimia which invariably leads to not menstruating for long periods of time.

There are ways of preventing osteoporosis and certainly in my practice over the years the elimination of allergens, the foods that trigger the production of bradikinin,(a pain transmitting hormone,) a healthy balanced diet, meat, fish, fruit and vegetables, gentle healthy exercise, walking, swimming or cycling and the ingestion of proper balanced supplementation have proved invaluable. There is a myth that bone loss cannot be restored, it is certainly my experience and that of many hundreds of patients that it can. For women over the age of 35 and men over the age of 45 I recommend taking B-Alive starting with lx3td after food for a month and then decrease to 2 daily for the rest of their lives. NAG one morning and night will help to repair intercartilagenous joints and intervertebral disc spaces. Three to six months is usually sufficient to correct the problem.

Good luck and good health.

Gwynne. H. Davies
Clinical Ecologist

B-Alive available from Hildreth & Cocker 0181675 2755.

NAG available from Biocare Ltd 0121433 3727.

Books and articles referenced for rheumatism and arthritis.

Overcoming Food Allergies. Gwynne.H. Davies.Pages 45 - 62.

Rheumatism and Arthritis - Jayson & Dixon. Pan.1974.

Arthritis,Rheumatism and Psoriasis.- Jan De Vries. Mainstream Publishing. 1986.

Goodbye to Arthritis - Patricia Byrivers - Century Arrow. 1985.

Say No To Arthritis- Patrick Holford - ION Press.I993.

Relief From Arthritis - John. E. Croft - Thorsons.1979.

A Doctors Proven New Home Cure for Arthritis - Giraud. W. Campbell. Parker.I972.

Arthritis and Common Sense - D.D. Alexander.Worlds Work Ltd. 1957.

The Practical Guide to Candida - Jane Mc Whirter. All Hallows Foundation